The Beginners Herbal Handbook

Contents

Introduction

I am constantly astonished by the power of these familiar, often humble plants. When our daughters have cuts and grazes to be dealt with, I dress them with a cool green Comfrey Ointment - or with a lotion made from the orange flowers of the common Marigold - knowing that pain will be soothed and healing rapid. Bedtime wakefulness and upset tummies have both alike been charmed away by Chamomile tea, colds have been nipped in the bud by a Mustard footbath, and doses of a fiery red concoction made from - amongst other things - Cayenne, Ginger and the creamy blossoms of the Elder.

Coughs have been loosened with Garlic Syrup and sore throats eased by a gargle of Sage. Herbal medicine is equally effective for more sophisticated woes: even the direst of hangovers has been known to yield to a fragrant tea containing Lavender Flowers, invented by a green-fingered country herbalist. And when my husband was convalescing from a serious operation three years ago, his recovery was speeded by a course of a herbal newcomer - a tonic course of *Eleutherococcus senticosus* or Siberian Ginseng, Russia's answer to the original Ginseng of China.

Herbal medicine in the home, however, is more than just first aid for minor ailments. It can be truly preventive, for some of the commonest items in a kitchen - Onions, Garlic, Thyme, Mint, Sage - can help ward off many a malady if they are in constant use. And modern scientific research - particularly in France over the last two or three decades – has fully justified the honoured place these aromatic plants have enjoyed for centuries both in folk medicine and in traditional cookery.

Garlic taken regularly will keep many infections, coughs and colds at bay, check high blood pressure, tone up the heart and the digestive system. Thyme and Rosemary have been shown in laboratory trials to have antiseptic powers at least equal, if not superior to, carbolic acid. Mint has uniquely calming powers in the digestive tract, Lemon helps your liver and kidneys function smoothly, Nutmeg is a natural tranquilliser, Caraway Seeds prevent flatulence, and Cloves are excellent for the circulation. So the housewife who adds these lively, aromatic flavours to her cooking, instead of serving up the bland products of the packaged-food industry, is giving her family more than just an extra-tasty meal.

Many of the plants commonly used in traditional medicine owe much of their value to their high content of vitamins and minerals. Yellow Dock, Burdock and Dandelion, used for centuries in blood-cleansing formulae, are all rich in the iron essential to good circulation. Skullcap, one of the best-known and most useful herbal sedatives, is high in calcium and magnesium, both vital to a healthy nervous system. Nettles - an old country remedy for anaemia as well as rheumatism – are rich in iron, silicon and potassium. Packaged in plants, these essential nutrients are easily assimilated by our bodies. Thus, herbal remedies can have a beneficial effect on our general health, as well as dealing with specific troubles.

The same could certainly not be said of many of the remedies sold over the chemist's counter or supplied on prescription. Antihistamines, corticosteroids, painkillers, tranquillisers, sleeping tablets, antibiotics, even the common aspirin which is swallowed so often and so unthinkingly, can all have side-effects ranging from quite mild to seriously damaging, even life-threatening.

In the case of small children, I find this particularly tragic. Given a good diet and plenty of exercise, children are naturally lively, healthy creatures, who will shake off their childhood coughs, colds and fevers with a minimum of trouble most of the time. Yet I know of many children who have courses of antibiotics at the first sign of a sore throat or upset stomach, aspirin every time they complain of an aching head, paracetamol for their colds, and spoonfuls of quite powerful sedatives if they can't get to sleep at night. Such children rarely: seem to enjoy sturdy health - how can they build up their own natural powers of resistance? The French healer Maurice Messegue suggests that children who rarely, if ever, receive medicine, other than the mildest of simple herbal remedies, respond much faster to much smaller doses of antibiotics when a time comes that they are desperately needed. And, in my own experience, I've found that on the very rare occasions we give our children aspirin, just half of one seventy-five mg 'Junior' tablet is effective, although the suggested dose for children over eight is between four to eight tablets.

Drugs are among the chemical pollutants with which our bodies are today continually - and unavoidably - bombarded: thousands of additives in every item of processed food, pesticide and insecticide residues in the fruit and vegetables we eat, dozens of different chemicals unthinkingly used in domestic cleaning products or gardening aids, traces of

chlorine, of toxic metals like lead or cadmium in the air we breathe and the water we daily drink, all these add up to massive stress for our immune systems, and our adaptive powers. The enormous increase in such allergic symptoms as depression, fatigue, migraine, eczema, asthma, and hay fever is one result of this mounting burden of environmental pollution.

We cannot choose the air we breathe, nor completely avoid the chemical contamination of our food and water, but we can at least use for our medicine the natural substances to which our bodies have adapted for hundreds of thousands of years.

In this book I have collected together dozens of simple herbal remedies for the everyday aches and pains and woes which afflict us at one time or another. I have deliberately selected remedies with a long and proven history of safe use.

They are mild, gentle and - in the doses I have suggested – can have no harmful side-effects. Where any degree of caution needs to be used, I've said so. Some people, for instance, find

Garlic irritating to their intestinal tract, and Arnica, even highly diluted, applied externally, and has been known to cause a rash on some super-sensitive skins. There are other cautions I have dealt with in a separate section immediately preceding the main 'Ailments' section, but in general you can use these remedies with confidence, knowing that even if they do not bring about a marked improvement, at least they are doing you no harm.

Some of the ailments for which I have suggested remedies are so minor that people wouldn't think of bothering their doctors about them - colds, bruises, cuts and sores, hangovers, the odd headache or upset stomach, the occasional sore throat.

This work, however, is certainly not intended as a guide to the diagnosis and treatment of major illness. Disorders of the heart, liver, kidneys and so on, are far too serious for home doctoring: they should be referred to a professional practitioner without delay. So; obviously, should acute infectious diseases, especially in children.

There are certain symptoms, too, which could indicate a serious medical problem, and for which professional advice should be sought without delay: persistent headaches, mild but persistent fever, recurring pains in the stomach, bowels or elsewhere, blood in your urine or stools, unaccountable weight loss, chronic coughing or indigestion, vaginal bleeding between periods.

I have, however, suggested remedies which can help alleviate pain and discomfort in certain serious problems, once they have been diagnosed - cystitis, colitis, hepatitis, gastric ulcers - and which can safely be taken even if you are receiving medication from your family doctor. And in the case of infectious diseases, there are simple herbal remedies which can help enormously to stimulate the body's defence mechanisms, combat infection, and rebuild health once the fever has passed.

I have also suggested remedies for several painful chronic conditions - for instance, arthritis, bronchitis, skin disorders - because many of the people suffering from them, once their condition has been diagnosed by their family doctor or a specialist, are anxious to try a herbal remedy to see if it can bring the relief and improvement that modern drugs so often fail to supply.

I cannot emphasise too strongly however that, while even simple herbal remedies - such as are mentioned here – can often bring about a marked improvement in such cases, a trained professional herbalist should be consulted where this is possible. Not only can he draw on a far wider range of effective herbs, with long experience and training to guide him, but like other practitioners of natural medicine, he will carefully study the patient's medical history, diet and lifestyle, rather than simply prescribe for the relief of symptoms. He can then treat the underlying disorder, aiming to restore the patient to full health.

Note: The purist may regret that I have given the common English names of the herbs mentioned in this book rather than their correct botanical style - Marshmallow, for example, rather than *Althaea officinalis*. I have done so because this is the normal practice of herbal commerce in this country, although professional herbalists - and homoeopathic chemists _ use the botanical names.

About Herbal Medicine

A seventeenth-century apothecary made up herbal remedies in dozens of different forms - elixirs, boluses, cordials, cataplasms, plasters, syrups - and many of these names, although no longer in general use, linger on in herbals, to confuse and alienate the modern reader. Some of the names of plants used sound like mediaeval mumbo-jumbo – False Unicorn Root, Blessed Thistle, Lesser Galangal. The terminology of herbal medicine can be confusing too, although once you get to know the meaning of words like diaphoretic (perspiration inducing), demulcent (soothing) and carminative (relieving flatulence and colic), they're a useful shorthand way of indicating how a particular plant is used.

Those new to herbal medicine are often puzzled by what seems like the large number of herbs in a single formula, including some that sound most unlikely: why do you keep seeing Capsicum or Cayenne Pepper, for heaven's sake?

The reason for adding more than one herb is that more than one action is usually desired. Herbal formulae for rheumatism, for instance, are usually designed to promote the elimination of toxic wastes from the system, so they may include herbs with a diaphoretic action, such as Yarrow or Guaiacum, herbs with a diuretic action (increasing the quantity of urine), such as Bearberry or Clivers, and herbs with a laxative action such as Rhubarb. They will certainly include a herb with an anti-inflammatory and anti-rheumatic action, such as Willow. And most formulae contain a small amount of a highly stimulating herb, such as Cayenne or Ginger, to warm and energise the entire system, and give your circulation a boost, so that the herbal remedy has a real chance to work.

Most herbs have more than one action. Yarrow, for instance, is both a useful stimulant and a diuretic into the bargain and the herbal practitioner in composing a prescription will be careful to choose herbs that interact with and reinforce each other. Where particularly powerful herbs are used, which might have a locally irritating effect on body tissue; he may add a demulcent or calming herb to balance their action. For example soothing Liquorice is often added to diuretic formulae.

Some combinations of herbs are as classic as bacon and eggs: the diaphoretic, warming mix of Elder Flowers, Peppermint and Yarrow, for instance, is recommended for the onset of chills and winter fevers. Of six or seven herbs the practitioner might choose for one action, there may be two, or three that work exceptionally well together, and are constantly combined.

Every practitioner, too, has his own favourites. Some of the most successful formulae have been copied and handed down through several generations of herbal practice, and are now enshrined in commercial remedies- Potter's Tabritis tablets for arthritis, for instance.

From all this it should be evident that making up a successful herbal formula is an art for the expert - just as devising a successful new dish is an art for the master chef: both are beyond the scope of the amateur.

Fortunately, as the pages of this book show, there are dozens of excellent formulae available in made-up form, so that even if you are unable to consult a herbal practitioner, you can still benefit from this level of professional skill. Moreover, single-herb infusions are perfectly satisfactory for many of the minor or transitory ailments mentioned in this book, and work extremely well.

How to Prepare Herbal Remedies

There are several bits and pieces it is useful to have when preparing herbal remedies. One of them is a proper herbal infuser: an 8 oz (225 ml) china cup with a perforated china strainer inside it, and a close-fitting lid, for making your herbal infusions one dose at a time. An old-fashioned inhaler with a spout, for lung-cleansing and soothing inhalations of aromatic herbs, is very handy too. And I wish somebody would present me with a set of pretty dark green jars with tightly fitting lids and decorative labels, for storing my dried herbs.

None of these is essential, though. You can keep a small china teapot especially for your herbal infusions, or even make them in a mug with a plate on top. A wide-necked jug - plus a ' towel to drape around your head - can be used for inhalations.

Old jam or coffee jars with screw-top lids can be used for storing herbs and they should be kept in a cool dark cupboard, away from light. ,

There's nothing complicated, either, about the herbal remedies I've suggested you try making up. They come in four forms;

The Infusion

What are charmingly known as the 'aerial' parts of the medicinal plant - flowers, leaves, stems, or all three, known collectively as the 'herb' as opposed to its root - are usually prepared by infusion. A teaspoon of the dried herb – double the quantity if you are using fresh - is put in an infuser, mug, or small teapot. A cupful of water, just on the boil, is poured on to it, and it is then covered - since much of the herb's therapeutic value may be in its volatile oils, which would be lost through evaporation - and left to steep for at least ten minutes. It is then strained. Proper herbal infusers have their own built-in strainers. Otherwise, you could buy the one-cup size of the Melita coffee filters, and strain your infusion through a filter-paper. Keep the filter specially for herbs, though - some of them might give the next cup of coffee an odd taste. Infusions to be used as an eyewash should always be strained through a paper, in this way, or alternatively through a piece of muslin. Herbal infusions can be sweetened to taste with honey. They are usually drunk warm, and taken in this dose - which should be a smallish cupful after straining – three times a day, usually before meals. Unless otherwise specified. all herbal infusions mentioned in this book are made in this way.

If you wish, you may make up a larger quantity, enough for a day's dosage, by adding a pint of water (550 ml) to one ounce (30 g) of the herb. After the first dose, the remainder should be covered and stored in the refrigerator, and gently reheated for use in a covered glass or enamel - not aluminium - pan, without boiling. It's unwise to store infusions longer than twelve hours.

More and more of the classic medicinal herbs are now being packaged in handy teabag form, so that you can make up your herbal remedy with as little fuss as an ordinary cup of tea. The Greither's Floradix range from the German manufacturer Salus includes such useful herbs as Vervain, Thyme, Yarrow, Sage and Orange Blossom, as well as old favourites like Chamomile, Lime Blossom and Peppermint; they're made from pharmacopoeia-quality herbs in 2 g bags - a useful dose.

Many of Potter's old-established and popular Compounds are now available in tea-bag form too, packed in canisters of twenty: among them their Nervine Herbs for Nervous Debility and Irritability, Kasbah Remedy for backache and urinary disorders, and Sciargo for the treatment of sciatica and lumbago.

The Decoction

The roots of a medicinal plant are usually stronger medicine than its flowers and leaves, though they may have a similar action, and they take correspondingly longer to extract. I have suggested very few remedies for making up from roots, because it's that much messier and more fuss. But it's still quite simple, and, for most herb roots this is how you do it.

One ounce of the root (30 g) is placed in a glass or enamel pan and one pint (550 ml) of cold water poured over it. Bring to the boil, then turn the heat down and simmer for about half an hour. Then Strain.

Poultices

For years poultices were consigned to oblivion by orthodox medicine, as more fashionable pills and injections took their place. But we are fast learning, through modern science, how efficiently certain substances, particularly volatile plant oils, can be absorbed through the skin and diffused through the system without undue irritation of the digestive tract. So poultices are making a comeback as an excellent way of getting a local effect fast - and indeed, those who practise herbal medicine have never stopped using them. Poultices sound messy and complicated: in fact, they couldn't be simpler. They are most commonly used for abscesses and other local inflammations. Powdered Comfrey Root, Marshmallow Root, or Slippery Elm Bark are the three used most often. (Buy them in powdered form: crushing your own is tricky.) A tablespoonful of the powder is moistened with hot water -better still with a herbal tea such as Comfrey Leaf, or Chamomile - till it's a thick paste. Smear this on pieces of sterile lint, fold another piece over it, and apply it to the inflamed area as hot as can be borne. Renew it when it has cooled. Big Plantain or Comfrey Leaves, carefully washed first, can be wrapped around on top.

Compresses

Pieces of clean lint are moistened in a lotion made up of various herbs and applied to a bruised, inflamed or injured area. They can be loosely bandaged into place if you want to keep them on longer. Herbs also come in the form of Liquid, or Fluid Extracts, which are the result of commercial heating, pressing or distilling processes which result in a highly concentrated form of the plant; and Tinctures, where the therapeutic properties of the plant have been extracted in diluted alcohol or glycerine.

Fluid Extracts and Tinctures are used by professional herbalists for obvious reasons of convenience, but for the amateur, calculating dosages becomes tricky, and even small quantities of either probably represent more of anyone herb than is likely to be needed by one household or person, although I have listed one or two in this book.

For suggestions on how to equip a family first-aid cupboard, see the separate section at the end.

Taking Herbal Medicines: Some Do's and Don'ts

Many of the herbs used as home remedies can work as fast as any modern synthetic drug to bring relief for minor aches, pains or ailments - sore throats, boils, gastric upsets, scalds, bruises, etc. But in the treatment of chronic disorders such as rheumatism or bronchitis, the action of medicinal herbs is slow, gentle and cumulative, working to strengthen and stimulate the various systems of the body over a long period of time.

So if you are taking a herbal remedy for a chronic condition, you should realise that although you can expect to feel some relief within two or three days, its full effect may not be felt until you have been taking it for a fortnight or longer. Invest in a course sufficient to last at least a month, to give it a fair trial: a single dose or a couple of tablets certainly won't do much lasting good.

How long should you go on taking a herbal remedy?

Most of the remedies I have mentioned in this book are fairly - mild, and in some cases - as with remedies for rheumatism and other chronic conditions - can be safely taken over long periods without risk, in the doses suggested here or by their suppliers.

No herbal treatment, however, should be seen as a substitute for the efficient working of your body's own natural defence system. The best herbal remedy in the world cannot do much, in the long term, for- somebody who is undermining his or her health by inadequate diet, too little exercise and excessive stress and tension.

Once you feel that the condition for which you are taking a herbal remedy is much improved, you should try tapering off the dose very gradually - instead of six tablets a day, take five a day for one week; then four, and so on. If your condition worsens, return to the original dose and try to reduce it again later. You may find that you can get it down to a maintenance dose of, perhaps, a tablet a day, or just an occasional one.

It's a good idea, too, from time to time, to have a day with no tablets at all, to give your body a chance to exercise its own healing powers unaided.

How safe is herbal medicine?

Most of the herbal remedies mentioned in this book are perfectly mild and safe, if used in the doses suggested either in this book or by their suppliers.

Do not make the common mistake of assuming, however, that because herbal medicine is perfectly safe and free from side effects when used with care, any number of herbal remedies can be swallowed with impunity. Just like any other food, drink or drug we take into our bodies, they can be abused if taken in excess. These are some of the more obvious problems:

Herbs with a very marked diuretic or laxative effect, such as those used in blood-cleansing formulae, should be taken in short courses of perhaps a week at a time, or they may end by depleting the body's vital forces rather than stimulating them.

Too many stimulating herbs, in turn, can be dangerous for someone with high blood pressure, though perhaps the only one in common use likely to give real trouble is Ginseng.

Herbs with a marked action on the heart should only be taken on professional advice: many herbs - among them Lily of the Valley, Hawthorn and Mistletoe - have a distinct effect on the blood pressure and could be dangerous when self administered, particularly if you are taking other medication at the same time.

Herbal nerve tonics, anti-depressants and tranquillisers may not be 'addictive' in the full clinical sense of the world, but even psychological dependence on a herbal remedy, however free from side effects', is not a healthy state of affairs, and leaves the basic problem unresolved. A habit, as they say, is a habit. Indeed, the mere fact of a remedy's 'safety' may lull us into laziness. Endlessly relying on herbal laxatives – or tranquillisers, or digestive tonics - is much the same as relying on synthetic drugs.

Pregnant women are well advised to avoid all drugs - synthetic or herbal- except for the mildest of herbal teas, such as Peppermint, Lime or Chamomile, or those prescribed by a competent herbal practitioner. The exception is Red Raspberry Leaf tea which - taken during the last three months of pregnancy - can help to secure an easier delivery.

Essential oils are powerfully concentrated medicine: they should be used with great caution, only in the small amounts suggested.

There are several herbs, such as Buckthorn, Cascara, Poke Root or Blue Flag, which are fairly potent and can be toxic in overdose. They are perfectly safe when prescribed by a qualified herbal practitioner, or carefully balanced in long tried formulae licensed by the British Department of Health (look For the Product Licence number on the label), since the Department quite rightly tends to err on the side of caution.

But I would strongly and urgently advise against making your own home brews from such active herbs as these.

Garlic can be irritant to the digestive tract in some people, and nursing mothers should avoid it - it could give their babies colic.

.

High and regular intake of tannins is now being linked with cancer of the oesophagus, to which people who drink lots of black tea seem to be statistically more prone than those who like their tea with milk. Many herbs contain tannins, particularly those made from barks and roots, though most tannin-high herbs are those only used from time to time.

However, two tannin-containing teas likely to be drunk more regularly are Peppermint and Raspberry Leaf and frequent users should bear this in mind.

All in all, however, the safety record of herbal medicine is impressive even to its bitterest opponents, and the rare mishaps that occur are often due to mistakes in plant identity.

For instance the large distinctive leaves of the Foxglove - highly toxic - have been brewed up into teas in the belief that they were Comfrey, with near fatal results.

Comfrey: a special note
In the course of experiments ~n Australia within the last decade, .certain alkaloids were detected in the leaves of

Comfrey which, when experimentally fed in large quantities to a susceptible strain of rats, induced a liver cancer in some of them. As a result, Comfrey itself is now under a cloud. The

Department of Health has not ruled against the continued use of the herb. And most herbal practitioners and experts are convinced of the safety of this valuable herb, which has enjoyed so high a repute for so long, and "has been taken continuously for months and even years without any previous suggestion that it could be causing this kind of problem.

Experiments are now in progress to establish once and for all whether this suspicion ·is indeed an unjustified slur on the reputation of a wonderful herb. Meanwhile, however, the cautious may wish to avoid it, so I have suggested Comfrey mainly for external use, where its great healing powers could hardly be dispensed with.

Is it safe to take herbal medicine at the same time as the drugs your family doctor prescribes?

Generally speaking, there should be no problem with mild herbal teas, such as those taken to raise perspiration and stimulate the circulation in the early stages of a fever.

Demulcent herbs such as Marshmallow and Slippery Elm, that soothe inflammation of the mucous membrane, can safely - and indeed profitably - be taken with antibiotics aimed at countering infection, and might help neutralise undesirable side-effects; and most of the herbal remedies for rheumatism and arthritis can safely be taken in combination with the painkillers prescribed by doctors.

However, even mild herbs may interact with other drugs in ways you might not expect: or the two combined may produce too powerful an effect, such as taking herbal sedatives at the same time as barbiturates, or a herbal laxative as well as one prescribed by your doctor. So if you are in any doubt at all, check with a herbal practitioner: few doctors know a great deal about the constituents or physiological action of herbs, so they will probably err on the side of caution and advise against taking them.

Most people turn to herbal medicine because they don't feel they're getting much benefit from modern drugs; so it seems a little absurd to be taking both. But if you want to switch from one to the other, don't do so without consulting your doctor, or a herbal practitioner. This is very important, because the body can become 'hooked' on many drugs – including painkillers and tranquillisers and more importantly still, any drugs for a heart condition - if it has been taking them for a long time. So if you plan to try a herbal remedy, take professional advice before stopping a course of medication prescribed by your doctor, and only then start tapering off the drug; you can build up gradually to the full dose of the herbal remedy.

Is herbal medicine safe for children?

Certainly it is, when you're using mild herbal teas instead of powerful' drugs like aspirin, antihistamines and steroids - which many thoughtful family doctors today are unhappy about giving to children under ten or so. In my own experience, herbal medicine is more effective too, bringing swift relief and recovery in such various ailments as headache, sore throat, sleeplessness, nappy rash and colic.

(In this new revised edition, children's ailments, with their remedies, are now gathered together in a special section of their own.)

Getting the best out of herbal medicine

Herbs are splendidly effective medicine, but don't expect them to perform miracles. If you are run down from lack of fresh air and exercise, or not enough rest, or if your health is being steadily undermined by a poor diet low in the nutrients you need to keep healthy, vigorous and energetic, the most skilfully prescribed herbal medicine in the world will do little for you. So before you spend time, money and effort on herbs, it's worth pausing to consider, first, if you are doing everything else possible to promote your health, or cope with a particular problem. A healthy diet is high in fresh vegetables and fruit, often eaten raw; it includes whole grains, nuts and seeds, eaten while they are fresh and in good condition; and it is low in fat, particularly the animal fats. Sugar and white flour should be eliminated as far as possible and red meat eaten sparingly, or replaced by chicken, fish and vegetable protein.

Alcohol should be kept to a minimum, and tea and coffee replaced as often as possible by mild herbal teas. There are many attractive blends on the market today as well as favourite single-herb brews, and they come in instant tea-bag form. The famous blends of Celestial Seasonings from the United States are well-known, and there are now delicious home-produced blends too, such as the Secret Garden range from the London Herb and Spice Company.

Herbal remedies can bring magically fast relief from the pain or inconvenience of a headache, a digestive problem or a mild bout of diarrhoea. And often this kind of effective symptomatic relief is just what the sufferer wants, so that he or she can get on with life or continue to enjoy a holiday. But it can never be said too often that these trivial ailments are often the earliest warnings of more serious trouble, and if they recur or show signs of becoming chronic, it is time to start considering underlying causes, and to seek professional help.

Ailments A-Z

Acne

Acne occurs when the sebaceous glands that keep your skin lubricated become blocked. Excess sebum is then trapped beneath the skin surface, infection is readily set up, and the disfiguring pustules erupt all over the face of the sufferer.

Especially common in adolescence, it is often the result of hormonal imbalance. A lot of women, myself included, find that it vanishes for ever with the birth of their first baby. But stress, or bad diet leading to elimination problems, will certainly make it worse, while a careful diet, combined with a course of blood-cleansing herbs, may bring it completely under control. See Skin Problems for general advice. If home treatment is unsuccessful, consult a trained herbal practitioner.

Acne sufferers are often so desperate to attack those horrid spots that they forget all about the need to care for the skin in between them - which may be dry, sensitive, and desperately in need of a little tender loving care. Acne-ridden skin must be kept scrupulously clean at all times, but that doesn't mean harsh soaps or strongly astringent tonics. On the contrary, it is vital to preserve the delicate acid balance of your skin, and to use only the gentlest, mildest of preparations, made if possible strictly from natural ingredients. Fortunately, there are several such ranges now on the market, and most health food shops sell a selection. Names to look for include Blackmore, Rachel Perry and Faith Products. The Weleda Skin and Beauty Therapy range are made from natural ingredients such as essential oils, distilled Witch Hazel,

Grapefruit juice, Rosewater and Gum Tragacanth, Chamomile and Calendula. The Yin-Yang range is Ph. balanced, and includes a delicious-smelling face pack called Precious Earth, made from an acidic clay and extracts of seaweed, which is very gentle, but stimulating and deep-cleansing too.

Calendula - common Marigold - is a prime ingredient in many natural beauty products because of its effective healing and soothing powers.

Chamomile is equally soothing and purifying - infuse a teaspoonful of the dried heads, or a Chamomile teabag, in a cupful of boiling water, covered, for ten minutes. Strain, cool and apply in the same way. The flowering tops of Yarrow, Elder or Lavender are equally useful. Take a handful of the fresh or dried flowers and steep, covered, in a pint (550 ml) of boiling water for ten minutes, then strain, cool and use as a wash. Lavender is both antiseptic and very calming to the nerves: one of the essential oils in the Four Thieves' Vinegar made by Thornham Herbs is that of Lavender. Add a little of this to a cupful of an infusion of Yarrow flowers, to bathe infected areas. Finally, a bedtime Lavender bath - Weleda's Lavender Milk, for instance - will help to calm you, as well as your skin.

Very gentle steaming - be careful not to scald yourself – can help your skin to throw off impurities. Add a handful of any of the following herbs to a jug of boiling water: Chamomile to counter infection and inflammation, Lime Flowers or Sage Leaves to cleanse and purify, Thyme to stimulate and disinfect. Close your pores and cool your skin afterwards with a mixture of Rosewater and Witch Hazel.

The great temptation of the luckless acne sufferer is to pick and squeeze the pustules. The result is rapidly spreading infection and unsightly pitting and scarring. If you have succumbed to this temptation, make up a lotion of Tincture of Calendula or

Tincture of Hypercal- a few drops in a small cup of water - to dab the oozing pimple and then to bathe your face in case you've spread infection.

'Ripe' pustules can be safely brought to a head by poultices of powdered Comfrey Root. Take a teaspoonful and mix it to a paste with hot water or Comfrey tea, then spread it over the worst affected parts. Leave it on for as long as possible. Wash it off with a tea made from Comfrey Leaves - and use more of the same tea as a healing wash for ravaged and scarred skin.

Comfrey contains allantoin, which has the remarkable power of stimulating cell proliferation to encourage fast healing. Freshly squeezed lemon juice is bactericidal, cooling and stimulating to the blood. Paint it gently onto inflamed areas.

Arthritis *see* Rheumatism.

Allergies

Any herbal practitioner will confirm to you that the whole range of ailments with an allergic origin is massively on the increase today. 'Very few of the patients I see nowadays *don't* have allergic problems', one herbalist told me. Herbal remedies may not be able to clear the basic problem, but they can supply effective relief for tiresome or painful symptoms, and by promoting general health can reduce the body's susceptibility to allergies.

The range of ailments which can be triggered by common foodstuffs such as milk, wheat or oranges, or by exposure to chemicals such as artificial food colourings, the propellants in an aerosol spray, gas or petrol, seems almost limitless. And if there is a history of hay fever, asthma, eczema or migraine in your family - the' classic' allergy diseases - or if you yourself suffered from childhood bouts of colic, diarrhoea or eczema. It's wise at least to consider the possibility that your particular health problem may have an allergic origin. This is particularly true of diseases of the respiratory or digestive tract. The same herbalist told me of a woman who had had twenty-nine operations for blocked sinuses over the years, until a bright young locum she happened to see asked her if she had ever been checked for allergies. She had not. Since milk is a very common allergen, he suggested that she cut out milk and dairy products. Five days later, she found her sinuses beginning to drain properly for the first time in years. Herbal treatment helped repair the massive damage inflicted on her scarred and ravaged mucous membranes, and today, avoiding dairy products, she is perfectly well.

Conventional treatment for allergy problems is simply to eliminate the allergen as far as possible. But treatment by a skilful herbal practitioner can often get to the root of the problem by strengthening and toning the nerves, the digestive tract or the immune system of the patient, once the specific allergen has been identified; and in many cases allergies will then diminish in severity, or even disappear for good. Plenty of exercise to strengthen the immune system, and a healthy diet are vital to the success of such treatment. Raw foods - fruit, vegetables, nuts, seeds, sprouted grains, - are reported to be particularly valuable in training the body to overcome its allergic susceptibilities.

Warning: If the symptoms which have bothered you clear up after four or five days of avoiding a suspected allergen, be very cautious about re-exposing yourself to it, since your body will be even more sensitive to it. Dr Richard Mackarness, one of the pioneers of allergy treatment in this country, suggests having ready alkaline salts bought from the chemist in preparation, made from two parts of sodium bicarbonate to one of potassium bicarbonate. If after re-exposure your reaction is a severe one, drink a glass of water to which you have added two heaped teaspoons of these salts, followed by a glass of plain water. This will help 'switch off' the reaction. If your problem is asthma, or a psychological one such as depression, re-exposure should only be tried under the supervision of a doctor trained in clinical ecology.

Anorexia Nervosa

An eating disorder found typically in teenage girls, who become obsessed with the belief that they are overweight: the idea of eating thus becomes progressively more and more threatening. An allied eating disorder is *bulimia,* when they will go on eating binges, but deliberately induce vomiting afterwards. Conventional treatment is by psychotherapy, and, when the weight dips dangerously low, by hospitalisation and a programme of supervised high-calorie feeding to reverse weight loss. Professor Bryce-Smith of Reading University has found that this bizarre and increasingly common disorder may be due to simple deficiency of zinc, for which teenage girls have extra high needs for growth and hormonal reasons, and in which their diets easily become dangerously deficient when they start slimming, or eat poor junk foods. He suggests a simple and inexpensive way to test if this is the case: get your chemist to make up a solution of 13.2 g of zinc sulphate heptahydrate and distilled water, adding more distilled water to make up a litre 5-10 mls of this, swirled around the mouth, will be completely tasteless to those deficient in zinc, although nauseatingly strong and repellent in taste to those well supplied. A 5 ml spoonful in half a cup of water will supply 15 mg of elemental zinc: anorexics will probably need at least this dose, three times daily, taken at mealtimes; higher doses may be needed to obtain a clinical response - even two or three times this amount. In most cases, the response will be dramatically swift, but zinc supplementation should be continued till weight is normal again. If the anorexia is already severe and the patient undergoing medical treatment you must make certain the doctor knows about and agrees to this treatment. Even then, anorexics may relapse if they stop taking the zinc, for which they may have extra-high need, and they may need a maintenance dose of it daily indefinitely.

Months or years of poor nutrition mean that even when cured, anorexics and bulimics may well have digestive problems of one kind and another - see under Digestive Problems. Their diet needs to be extra healthy, rich in such nutritious foods as oats, whole grains, nuts and seeds, to supply the Vitamins A and B6 needed for maximum absorption of zinc, raw vegetable salads, plenty of fruit. If they are vegetarian, as so many teenagers are these days, they should be aware that meat is the most reliable source of zinc in our diets, and plan their menu accordingly. The black coffee to which so many anorexics and bulimics become addicted should be cut to a minimum. It is very bad for both nerves and digestion in large quantities.

Asthma

The chesty wheezing, the difficulty in expelling air, the painful tightness of the diaphragm, and the struggle to breathe are all familiar symptoms of asthma. They may be due to inflammation of the mucous membrane lining the small air passages, which then swell, making breathing more difficult, or to a spasm of the diaphragm or the muscles in the bronchial area, which then constricts the air passages to produce the same effect. Mucus accumulates, and the spasm makes it difficult to cough this away. Acute attacks may be due to the air passages becoming blocked by accumulations of dried mucus. Chesty colds and bronchial infections will also trigger attacks in those with asthmatic tendencies. The two most likely causes of asthma are emotional tension, producing this particular effect 'in asthma sufferers, or an allergic reaction, triggered either by certain foods - particularly those containing chemical additives - or to atmospheric pollutants such as house dust, pollen etc. (See also the section on Allergies.) Poor diet, little or no exercise, and not enough fresh air, all contribute to the build-up of catarrhal mucus, and undermine general resistance. Often simply improving your diet by cutting out junk foods and stepping up your intake of fresh fruit, vegetables and whole grains, together with regular exercises which improve breathing (yoga is particularly good), will result in a steady improvement.

There are many herbs which are useful both in dealing with the underlying causes of asthma, and treating its more painful symptoms. If your asthma is chronic or severe (and cardiac asthma, which is a different problem with similar symptoms, has been ruled out), you should consult a herbalist who can prescribe the treatment best suited to your particular problem. In milder cases, try the following suggestions.

Chronic asthma sufferers should fill their gardens or window boxes with such aromatic herbs as Thyme, Marjoram, Pine, and Lavender. The volatile oils of these plants contain substances which not only can help to disinfect and soothe inflamed mucous membrane, attacking local infection, but also to relax the muscles. Thyme, Marjoram and Lavender can all be infused, covered, in boiling water, strained and sweetened with a little honey and drunk hot to bring relief during attacks. Hot compresses on the chest will also help - volatile oils penetrate the skin very quickly. Another way to obtain the benefit of these useful aromatic plants is to make a particularly strong infusion of Eucalyptus, Pine, Rosemary,

Lavender, Thyme or Marjoram, and pour it into a hot bedtime bath.

There are plants that help to break down accumulated mucus, and encourage a cough to clear it from the air passages.

A useful one is Hyssop. Add a teaspoon of the dried herb to a teacupful of water, infuse covered for ten minutes, then strain. A little honey can be added. Drink three times a day, or during attacks.

Asthma triggered by a bronchial infection can be helped by any of the herbs mentioned under Bronchitis.

During attacks', a few drops of Potter's Antispasmodic Drops in a small glass of warm water may bring relief.

Potter's Asthma & Chest Mixture helps to tone and cleanse the bronchial tubes.

Gerard House Lobelia Inflata Compound Tablets contain the queen of the antispasmodic herbs - Lobelia – together with Gum Ammoniacum, Cayenne, Capsaicin, to stimulate and tone the whole system, and Squills, which are both stimulating and help to clear mucus. Lobelia is used in another formula, first compounded by a herbalist in 1860: Napier's Lobelia Herb Syrup contains Lobelia, Capsicum, Aniseed, Camphor and Blood-root.

The Bio-Strath Thyme Formula combines this particularly useful plant with Primula, which their researches showed to be even more effective in countering inflammation and pain than the

Willow Formula. The tonic base of Bio-Strath will help to improve general resistance. (See Convalescence.)

See also Bronchitis *and* Nerves.

Athlete's Foot

Athlete's foot is spread by a little burrowing fungus which loves the warm, moist skin between your toes. It thrives in locker rooms and gym changing rooms. Wearing socks and shoes made of sweaty synthetics and not drying properly between your toes encourage it to settle in for a long stay. To avoid it, keep your feet scrupulously clean and dry, use a mild foot powder, wear socks with a high proportion of cotton in them, and leather or canvas shoes. There are a number of ways to get rid of it. Make a fairly strong tea from Goldenseal Root and swab between your toes. '

Thyme is a powerful disinfectant and fungicide. Heat fresh Thyme leaves in a little oil until they have lost their colour, then apply the strained oil. An alternative is to use the essential oil of Thyme, or to make a double-strength infusion from the fresh or dried leaves, and bathe the feet in it.

Rosemary can be used in the same way.

Make a strong infusion of Agrimony and bathe the feet in it, swabbing between the toes.

Wash your feet in hot soapy water, and then apply Garlic Oil between the toes.

Soak your feet in a footbath to which you have added a little of Weleda's Rosemary Bath.

A couple of drops of the Essential Oil of Lavender, rubbed into the affected bits, sometimes clears the condition.

See also Feet *and* Skin Problems.

Bad Breath

If you have persistent bad breath, either you have a dental problem .which needs urgent attention - decaying teeth or infected gums - or your digestive system is in poor shape, in which case see Digestive Problems. For suggestions on keeping your gums firm, clean and healthy, see Gums.

Meanwhile, here are some suggestions for sweetening your breath.

Boil a good sprig of Thyme in a cupful of water for two or three seconds. Then leave it to steep, covered, for ten minutes.

Use half the water as a mouthwash, swishing it around between your teeth; drink the other half.

Make an infusion of Rosemary Leaves and Flowers by pouring a cupful of boiling water over a teaspoon of Rosemary. Cover and leave to infuse for ten minutes. Use half as a mouthwash and drink the rest. Both Thyme and Rosemary, incidentally, are first-class antiseptic and firming treatments for your gums, as well as excellent tonics for the digestion.

Make an infusion of Lavender Flowers by boiling a teaspoonful in a cup of boiling water for two minutes. Leave to steep, covered, for ten minutes. Drink between meals.

Make a cup of Peppermint tea - with a teabag or by infusing a teaspoonful of fresh or dried leaves in a cupful of boiling water, covered. Add a little freshly squeezed Lemon juice, and drink.

Chew fresh Parsley, or fresh Mint leaves.

Boils & Abscesses

A tendency to boils suggests that you are run down, or that you suffer - perhaps without even realising it - from some degree of constipation, and that toxic wastes are accumulating in the bowels. Take plenty of exercise to improve your circulation, and check under Constipation if that could be the problem. For general advice, see under Skin Problems.

Meanwhile, you have a nasty boil - or several. Here are some useful remedies for coping with it.

Bind on a slice of Lemon to bring it to a head, or paint on neat Lemon juice. Or moisten the square of gauze in an ordinary adhesive plaster with lemon juice and apply.

An Onion baked till soft, and applied as hot as you can bear it will help draw it to a head.

So will a poultice made from a teaspoonful of crushed Fenugreek Seeds (wrap them in foil, and use a rolling-pin): simmer them for 10 minutes, covered, in a cupful of water.

Strain, and apply the seeds on a piece of lint lightly bandaged into place. Don't throw the tea away: it's a lovely tonic drink, and will help break down build-ups of mucus throughout your system - which could be contributing to the problem in the first place.

If the boilis at the tip of a finger - a whitlow - the easiest way to apply the lemon cure is to make a hole in the side of a lemon and stick your finger into it - perhaps when you have a few lengthy telephone calls to make!

For other poultices - and how to treat the boil when it comes to a head and bursts - see under Abscesses, below. In either case, remember that cleanliness is vital: well-scrubbed hands, boiled water and sterilised lint dressings are essential.

Abscesses

Abscesses occur for much the same reasons as Boils - so act accordingly. If the abscess is hot, acutely painful and much inflamed, seek professional advice - particularly if you're running a temperature. (See Fever.) For milder cases, here are some suggestions:

Start taking a course of Echinacea straight away - a marvellous plant antibiotic, and a powerful blood-cleanser. One of the handiest forms in which to take this is Echinaforce, from Dr Vogel' s Bioforce range: a tincture of the fresh plant - herb and roots, to be taken several times daily, 10-20 drops in a glass of water. Potter's, Baldwin's and Gerard House also have Echinacea Tablets - the usual dose is one three times a day: or you can buy the dried root, and make a decoction, simmering one ounce of it (30 g) in one pint of water (550 ml) for 25 minutes.

See also Ulcers: External

Breast Feeding Problems

If the problem is insufficient milk, some of the fragrant warming spices that we use in the form of seeds can help.

Crush a teaspoon of Fennel seeds, pour a cupful of boiling water over them, cover and leave too steep for ten minutes.

Strain off the liquid and drink. Sweeten with a little honey, if liked.

Anise, Caraway, Cumin, Dill and Fenugreek can all be used in the same way. As well as helping with breast feeding problems, they are stimulating and warming herbs which will work to counter the low spirits and listlessness which can signal post-natal depression.

Vervain is another useful herb, equally effective for stimulating milk flow and lifting post-natal blues. Infuse a teaspoonful in a cup of boiling water, steep for ten minutes and drink three times a day. Vervain is now available in teabag form, in the Greither's Floradix range.

For sore, cracked nipples, Weleda's Calendula Ointment is magically soothing and healing. (It is now being used in the maternity wards of several hospitals near the Weleda gardens and factory in Derbyshire.)

To dry up milk flow, make up an infusion of half a teaspoonful of Sage in a cup of boiling water, and drink three times a day.

Bronchitis

There are many herbs that are effective in dealing with bronchitis, that painful, irritating infection of the bronchial tract. Among .the best known are Lungwort, White Horehound, Liquorice, Senega, Elecampane, Marshmallow, often used all together, with a pinch of Cayenne to' activate them and stimulate the circulation - a sort of herbal shot in the arm. These herbs get to work in two ways on your bronchitis: they will soothe inflamed and irritated tissue, and they will help to break up and expel the thick deposits of mucus which prompt the typical chesty bronchial cough. Some of them, such as Elecampane, are powerful bactericides as well; others have an antispasmodic effect, relaxing tense, contracted bronchi and alveoli - Lobelia, used by professional practitioners or in some licensed remedies, is outstanding in this respect. Others again will help to reduce the fever which accompanies even mild cases. For acute cases, seek expert advice.

Take half an ounce of Elecampane Root, simmer it in a pint of water for fifteen minutes. Strain, add a little honey and Lemon, both excellent for chesty ailments, if you like them, and drink warm, a cupful at a time, three times a day. For the irritating bronchitic cough, a particularly effective combination is White Horehound herb and Marshmallow Leaves. Mix them, and make an infusion of one teaspoon to a cupful of boiling water. Drink a wineglassful three times daily.

This is very effective with children. Sweeten it for them with a, little honey, and give them a dessertspoonful to a tablespoonful from time to time.

Lungwort, as you might expect, is a long-tried and trusted remedy, mildly diaphoretic, very soothing. Infuse a teaspoonful of the dried leaves in a cup of boiling water.

A friend of mine who was brought up in Spain still remembers the piercing, aromatic fragrance of Eucalyptus that filled the kitchen when the Spanish women brewed up their favourite remedy for his bronchitis. Take up to an ounce (30 g) of the dried leaves, put them in a pint (550 ml) of water, boil for a minute, then infuse closely covered for ten minutes.

Take three to five cups a day, warm. Very soothing - and a powerful bactericide.

The essential oils of several aromatic plants help bronchitis sufferers, either inhaled from a handkerchief or tissue on which you have sprinkled a few drops, or added to near-boiling water and inhaled, for two minutes at a time, three times a day.

Thyme, Pine, Eucalyptus, Lavender, Origanum are all effective. Inhalation of these volatile oils takes them directly into the lungs and bronchial tract where they are potent bactericides. Hospitals and many families still use the Tincture of Benzoin known as Friar's Balsam, and Olbas Oil combines several such oils, including Eucalyptus, Menthol, Peppermint and Wintergreen. A few drops of Olbas Oil can be rubbed into the back and chest of bronchial sufferers. Shirley Price's Coughs and Colds Treatment Oil can be used for inhalation, added to a bath, or added to a carrier oil for massage into neck and chest.

Another useful chest rub, if you and those around you can stand the smell, is made by chopping several cloves of Garlic very finely and adding them to equal parts of Vaseline. Warm them gently till the Vaseline has melted, stir, leave to cool and rub into chest and back, covering up warmly afterwards.

A wonderfully old-fashioned but highly effective remedy for chesty ailments is a Mustard poultice. Mix ordinary Mustard powder to a runny paste, with warm water: spread on a piece of lint, and apply to the chest, covering it up with a towel, until the skin has reddened slightly. Apply the poultice to several parts of the chest - back or front - and massage a little olive oil into the reddened part afterwards. This poultice stimulates local circulation to help counter inflammation.

Garlic is powerfully antiseptic and bactericidal - make an aromatic inhalation by crushing three or four cloves of Garlic and adding them to steaming hot water. Another method using

Garlic is to slice several cloves finely, put them in a jar, cover them with three or four tablespoons of runny honey, leave to stand covered for a couple of hours and then take teaspoonfuls of the resulting clear syrup at frequent intervals.

(I heard about this marvellous' remedy for years before I had the courage to try it out – I thought it must taste disgusting. In fact, it's oddly delicious, and my children take it without protest.)

Lobelia has such a powerful antispasmodic action that it's specific for asthma; the same qualities - plus its tonic effect on the entire respiratory system, and its expectorant action - make it excellent for bronchitis: Napier's of Edinburgh make a Lobelia Herb Syrup containing - as well as the Lobelia - Capsicum for its stimulant qualities, Blood foot for its expectorant action, Aniseed and Camphor - soothing and sedative. For the deep chesty cough of bronchitis, Napier's combine Lobelia with Gum Ammoniacum and Squill, both expectorants, and Cayenne and Capsaicin to stimulate circulation.

A sort of herbal 'catch-all' to suit all sorts of cough is Potter's Vegetable Cough Remover. The ingredients are:

Black Cohosh, Blood Root, Ipecac, Lobelia, Myrrh, Pleurisy Root, Skunk Cabbage, Comfrey, Coltsfoot, Elecampane, White Horehound, Hyssop, Skullcap, Valerian, Liquorice, Prickly Ash Bark, and Anise Oil. Between them, these useful herbs will counter infection, soothe inflammation, calm tension, aid expectoration, steady the irritable nerves of the sufferer, and stimulate their resistance. What more could you ask? Olbas Pastilles, sucked slowly, keep up a steady barrage of healing and disinfectant aromatic oils into the throat and lungs.

There are a number of excellent ready-made herbal remedies for bronchitis in tablet or liquid form. These are among the best.

Potter's Antibron Tablets contain an effective mixture of soothing, demulcent and expectorant herbs: Lobelia, Coltsfoot, Euphorbia, Liquorice, Pleurisy Root, Senega, Wild Lettuce, with a: dash of Cayenne.

Weleda's Sytra Tea contains Blackthorn Flowers, Iceland Moss, Elder Flowers, Marshmallow Root and Aniseed. Add a teaspoonful to a cup of boiling water, simmer for another two minutes, strain and sweeten with honey. Sip one to two cups slowly during the day.

Iceland Moss is a little lichen with marked soothing and expectorant properties - particularly effective at coping with the nausea that continued coughing can sometimes produce.

Gerard House combine it with a little Rhubarb and Lobelia in their- Iceland Moss Tablets. These are a particularly useful preventative for chronic sufferers.

Heath & Heather make a Heatherbron Cough Mixture containing Cubebs, Euphorbia, White Horehound, Sundew (a little bog plant especially good for respiratory ailments), Pleurisy Root, Senega, Lobelia, Liquorice, Squill, traces of Aniseed and Cayenne. -

To reduce the fever accompanying any bronchial infection, drink plenty of hot Elderflower or Yarrow tea, adding a little Composition Essence if you have it, or take a teaspoonful of Potter's E.P.C. in hot water three times a day.

Potter's Compound Herb 32, for Asthma and Bronchitis, is now available in canisters. of twenty teabags, and' contains some of the most useful' herbs to deal with painful, chesty conditions: Elecampane, Horehound, Hyssop, Irish Moss and Liquorice, with a dash of warming and stimulating Cloves.

See also Asthma, Coughs.

Bruises

If you bruise easily and badly, you may be deficient in Vitamin C, or your circulation may be poor. There are many excellent herbal remedies for bruises, though, which will allay the pain and halt the discoloration.

Before you do anything else, apply a hot compress (a cloth wrung out in hot water) to the affected part, to stimulate the circulation and relieve the pain. Follow this up with one of the treatments suggested below.

Swab it with Witch- Hazel- highly popular with children, who like its funny name and clean sweet smell. Smooth over it an Arnica Ointment: Weleda's or Nelson's. Make strong Comfrey tea, and apply as a hot compress. Smooth Comfrey Ointment or Comfrey Oil over it.

Make a lotion of cold water and a few drops of Tincture of Arnica. Apply as a cold compress. (Warning: Arnica is very toxic, and should never be used other than in diluted form and on unbroken skin. Some people with particularly sensitive skins may have a reaction to it.)

Bunions

Bunions are so evidently a self-inflicted woe that few books of home remedies, I find, bother even to mention them. But the inflammation of the distorted joint caused by years of ill fitting shoes can be very painful. Here are some ways to soothe it. See also under Chilblains; the same remedies will help bunions.

Paint fresh Lemon juice onto the bunion night and morning and leave to dry.

Paint Turpentine - the oily resin from some species of Pine trees - on to the bunion. (Synthetic "Turps" sold by D.I.Y. shops will not do.) Cover with lint and bandage lightly (to save the bedclothes).

Burns

Bad burns and scalds are a major medical emergency: summon professional help at once. Keep calm but act fast. It's what you do in the next few minutes, before the ambulance arrives, that could make the difference between serious injury or relatively minor damage. Your first priority is to cool the area of the burn as rapidly as possible, both to relieve the agony, and to stop further damage to tissue from the heat of the burn. If possible, immerse the burned part in cool - not ice-cold - water, and keep it there. If you have Tincture of Calendula, Hypericum or Hypercal to hand, add a few drops to the water, but get the burn into cool water first - don't waste time scouring the house for a mislaid medicine chest. If the burns involve chest, stomach or the whole body, wring out a large piece of clean linen - sheet or pillowcase - in cool but not ice cold water and wrap very gently round the burned area. In bad burns, the big danger is Shock. If the patient is unconscious, moisten his lips with a few drops of Dr Bach's Rescue Remedy or Potter's Antispasmodic Drops. If he can open his mouth and swallow, give him one of these - and then sips of water to drink with a touch of salt in it. When you have dealt with both heat and shock, cover the burn with clean - if possible, sterile lint, and keep the patient warm, comfortable and above all reassured until the ambulance arrives.

For minor burns and scalds, follow the same treatment.

When the burn is cooled, apply any of the following: Calendula Ointment, Weleda's Combudoron Ointment, Honey, Comfrey Ointment or Oil, cold Chamomile tea (use it for compresses) or a few drops of Oil of Lavender. '

See also Shock *and* Sunburn

Catarrh

Catarrh results from the irritation of the mucous membranes which line our air passages and digestive tracts. Where this membrane is irritated, it over-produces the watery mucus which normally lubricates and sterilises them. This, extra mucus thickens, settles - and causes problems. Nasal catarrh seems to be the most common, perhaps because it's the one that makes itself the most immediately obvious. But an unhealthy diet and even a mild degree of constipation which keeps toxic wastes circulating in your bloodstream will cause catarrh. (See Constipation, if this could be your problem.)

Another possible cause is allergy or sensitivity to certain foods. The commonest culprit - particularly in babies and children - is a milk allergy: thousands of people are susceptible without even knowing it. If you suspect this could be your case, simply drop all milk and dairy products from your diet for a week (but take supplements of calcium, and Vitamins A and D). If the catarrh is obviously better, you'll have to decide between life with catarrh or life without milk, butter and cheese. Babies and children need the calcium and protein provided by milk, so seek expert dietetic advice before experimenting. Persistent cases of catarrh should be seen by a herbal practitioner. Meanwhile, there are plenty of effective herbal remedies to alleviate the discomfort. A healthy diet with lots of fruit and fresh vegetables, together with regular open-air exercise, are the best possible prevention.

Take Garlic Oil Capsules - one three times daily. Add the juice of half a Lemon to half a pint of warm water. Snuff it very gently right up your nostrils several times a day.

This will make you sneeze and splutter like mad, but it will clear that heavy stuffed-up feeling, dispose of lurking streptococci, and leave you feeling marvellously light-headed.

It could also help to stop your catarrh developing into' Sinusitis or Earache.

For chronic catarrh, herbalists prescribe the leaves, stem and flowers of Hyssop, the fragrant blue-flowered perennial, useful for all respiratory ailments, since it soothes, heals and breaks up mucus. Infuse, covered, sweeten with honey and drink three times a day.

Slippery Elm and Marshmallow are other useful herbs - adding honey and Lemon juice will not only make them taste better but work better too.

The leaves and flowers of another pleasant garden herb, Borage, are also effective for catarrh. Infuse two teaspoons of the leaves and flowers in a cupful of boiling water.

Fenugreek tea, made by steeping a teaspoonful of the crushed seeds in a cupful of boiling water, covered, is a household remedy for catarrh and bronchial congestion in many parts of the world. Drink it freely. When the strained tea has cooled, you can also snuff it very gently up your nostrils to relieve congestion. Even chewing the seeds is helpful.

To clear that stuffed-up feeling, Weleda make a Catarrh Cream, containing, among other things, useful essential oils of Peppermint, Eucalyptus, and Camphor. Rub it all over your nose. Inhaling Olbas Oil from a handkerchief will also help to 'unblock' your head.

Potter's Antifect is so effective for catarrhal conditions that some family doctors are beginning to prescribe it. It's made from medicinal Charcoal- absorbent and antiseptic – Garlic and Echinacea.

Chilblains

If you have excellent circulation you won't have chilblains. In some people with poor circulation, who don't or can't keep their hands and feet warm, the small veins and arteries in their fingers and toes don't function efficiently, nerve endings become irritated and that itchy redness sets in. Plenty of exercise to improve your circulation, a healthy diet - with lots of dark leafy sprouting vegetables - will both help. To stop chilblains developing, or to soothe the itchy agony, here are some suggestions. Paint them with Lemon juice and let it dry on.

Apply a compress of finely grated Onion. Smooth in Calendula Ointment. Weleda's Frost Cream is made with Southernwood, Arnica, Balm of Peru and Rosemary Oil among other things - as well as a dash of petrol!

Oil of Lavender rubbed in is very soothing.

To improve your circulation generally, drink Buckwheat tea, made from the leaves and flowers of this cereal plant (a teaspoonful in a cup of hot water). It contains plenty of rutin to strengthen the small capillaries, and it will also help to lower high blood pressure.

Many familiar kitchen herbs and spices are tonics for the circulation - Black Pepper, Thyme, Marjoram, Garlic, Cumin, Cloves, Coriander, Cayenne and Ginger among them. So if you like spicy food with plenty of natural seasoning, indulge a healthy taste in winter.

Colds

In natural medicine, a cold is seen as the body's way of eliminating its toxic wastes in the form of mucous discharge when other means have broken down, or when the whole elimination system has been overloaded by faulty diet. We are much more susceptible to colds in winter, when we tend to eat heavier, starchy food, and less fruit, vegetables and salad. In this sub-healthy state, - which may equally be produced by unhappiness, or depression - viruses breed freely, and a cold unchecked may turn into influenza, bronchitis or even, in extreme cases, pneumonia.

At the very first sign of a cold you may just manage to thwart it by gently sniffing up your nostrils a mixture of warm water and lots of Lemon juice. If it's too late for prevention, herbal therapy follows classic sweat-it-out lines, aimed at eliminating toxins through your skin, and giving your body's immune system a healthy chance to fight back.

Hot Elder Flower tea, or Elder Flowers mixed with Yarrow herb, are tried and trusted country remedies. Put a teaspoonful in a cup, cover with boiling water and let them steep in a warm place for at least twenty minutes. Strain, add honey and drink as hot as possible before you go to sleep. If there's any left over, use it cold as a compress for the red eyes which so often signal a cold.

Hot Lemon and honey last thing at night is another good remedy and better still if you grate in some Ginger or Cinnamon. Almost all the warming aromatic spices are excellent for a cold, since they stimulate the circulation and encourage sweating. One of the most famous of all home herbal remedies, Composition Essence, formulated· by the dedicated herbalists of the nineteenth century, is made up of

Cayenne, Ginger and Cloves, and taken at the first sign of acute illness or fever - or the common cold. It's guaranteed to encourage healthy perspiration. Take a teaspoonful of it in a glass of hot water, sweeten with a little honey and drink it in bed, last thing at night, with the blankets piled on. The worst will be over by morning.

Another excellent way to ward off a cold is a Mustard footbath to be taken just before bedtime. Put a teaspoonful of ordinary yellow Mustard powder into a bucket or deep basin, add the same amount of household soda to soften the water, and add water to come halfway up the legs, as hot as can be borne.

Keep the feet in it for at least ten minutes or longer, topping it up with piping-hot water from time to time. Mop the feet dry, pull on thick socks and roll straight into bed.

Onions and Garlic are both so good for a cold that if you eat plenty of both all winter, you'll probably never get one - or if you do, it'll be a mild one-day affair. They're medicine as well as prevention, and food for the sickroom as well as medicine.

Simmer a big Onion in milk until its tender - about an hour then eat the softened Onion and drink the hot milk. If you really dislike the taste of Garlic, swallow Garlic Capsules instead.

If you have a Peppermint plant in your garden, pour a cupful of boiling water over a half a handful of the leaves: infuse covered for ten minutes; then drink the lovely bright green tea.

A very useful ready-made remedy is Potter's fiery E.P.C., a bright red mix of Elder Flower, Peppermint and Composition Essence, to be drunk a couple of teaspoons three times a day in hot water, one of them preferably at bedtime.

Olbas Oil with its blend of antiseptic aromatic oils can be exceptionally effective, and although the aroma is fierce at first, I find it disperses fairly fast. Sprinkle a few drops on a handkerchief and inhale. Alternatively rub a few drops of Olbas Oil into the throat, or sprinkle a few drops onto the pillow to be inhaled during sleep.

Cold Sores

These irritating, itchy, unsightly little blisters are the work of the *herpes simplex* virus, lying in wait in your system and flaring up from time to time in this exasperating form. If they're the 'persistent bane of your life, appearing every time you catch a cold, consult a qualified herbal practitioner, who can diagnose the underlying condition which makes you vulnerable, and treat it. For the cold sore, try any' of the following, painted on neat. Tincture of Myrrh, Tincture of Calendula, Spirits of Camphor, Pure Lemon juice or Honey.

Colic

The sharp stabbing pains in the stomach known as colic usually result from faulty digestion (see Digestive Problems). If they keep recurring, seek professional advice - they could be symptomatic of something more serious. Meanwhile, go to the spice rack for remedies:

Put a teaspoon of crushed Fennel Seeds in a cup, pour over them a cupful of boiling water, steep, covered, for twenty minutes. You can crush and add a few Cardamom Seeds to this mixture. Caraway Seeds are just as effective, prepared in exactly the same way.

So are Anise Seeds, and so is grated Ginger Root. And while you're waiting for your fragrant, spicy, comforting tea to be ready, sip plenty of warm water. Sometimes warm water alone can do the trick.

Peppermint tea is very soothing - use a teabag if you have one, or leaves from the fresh plant if you grow it. In the Middle East and all over Europe, mint tea is a highly popular after dinner drink - a delicious preventive medicine.

A drop of Peppermint essence, added to half a cup of hot water is another version of the same cure.

Peppermint tea is even better when combined with Lemon Balm. If you have any growing in your herb garden or kitchen window box, add a few leaves to the Peppermint before you pour on the boiling water, and infuse them together.

Colitis

When the mucous membrane lining your colon, or large intestine, becomes irritated and inflamed, the condition called

Colitis arises. There are two varieties - mucous and ulcerative - both equally unpleasant. Other dangerous diseases can give rise to the same symptoms, however, so it is essential to go to a doctor for a thorough diagnosis and check-up.

Allergies are a common cause of colitis, even the severest cases often responding almost magically to the simple removal of milk and dairy products from the diet (see Allergies) although of course other foods may be the culprit. Years of poor diet and little or no exercise can also contribute to this dangerous and life-threatening condition. (See Digestive Problems.) Conventional treatment has little to offer but antibiotics, to help control the bacterial infections that occasionally cause, and often follow, the problem, corticosteroids to give relief, and surgery. But herbal practitioners with their range of soothing, antiseptic, toning and healing plants are uniquely well equipped to deal with colitis.

They will advise you, too, on the changes in diet and eating habits that you will probably need to make in order to restore your colon to its normal healthy function. Meanwhile, the following remedies will help to soothe your damaged colon and allay the pain. (But none of these treatments should be used other than as interim measures - colitis is far too' serious a condition for experimental home treatment.)

Slippery Elm is particularly nutritious and soothing -.Add cold water to a teaspoonful of the powder to make a smooth, thin paste, then pour in a pint of boiling water, stirring all the time.

A little honey can be added.

Marshmallow Root is another great friend to the inflamed and irritated mucous membrane. On the instructions of a herbalist, I once gave some to a friend of mine in agonies of pain and diarrhoea from acute ulcerative colitis. Half an hour later the pain had subsided, and an hour later she ate some thick soup with a good appetite. -

Fenugreek can be an effective remedy for mucous colitis: soothing and emollient like Slippery Elm; it's combined with this useful bark in a Gerard House formula called Fenulin, in powder or tablet form. It also contains a little Turkey Rhubarb, Bayberry, and a dash of tonic Goldenseal.

See also Diarrhoea, Piles

Conjunctivitis

Conjunctivitis and Styes, particularly if they keep cropping up, are symptoms of poor general health or defective diet (see Skin Problems). Alternatively you may be feeling run down, overworked and tired. For a good tonic see Convalescence. If tiresome eye problems keep recurring, or don't yield to home treatment, seek expert advice and don't take chances. You can deal with the odd one yourself, as long as you remember that your eyes are precious and highly vulnerable to infection and re-infection. Both styes and conjunctivitis indicate the presence of bacteria, so scrupulous cleanliness is vital. Before you touch an infected eye, scrub your hands in soap and hot water, particularly under the nails. Use water that has been boiled - preferably pure bottled spring water - to sterilise eye baths, holding them with a pair of tweezers in the steam from a kettle and blotting them dry with a clean tissue. Don't use the same eyebath and lotion for both eyes: throw the lotion away and re-sterilise the eye bath before a second application. All this may sound like a lot of fuss: but as infection spreads very easily in the eyes, with potentially serious results, it is necessary. Any of the following make a good eye bath, soothing to inflamed tissue, healing and mildly disinfectant.

Use cool. Unused lotion may be kept covered in the refrigerator for not longer than a day.

A tablespoonful of Chamomile Flowers, steeped for twenty minutes in a cup of boiling water. Strain.

A teaspoon of Fennel Seeds, crushed, steeped, covered, for twenty minutes in a cup of boiling water. Strain. If you have a Chamomile teabag you can add it to the seeds before you pour on the water.

A tablespoonful of dried Elder Flowers, boiled for five minutes in a cupful of water, left to infuse for ten minutes, and strained.

Plain boiled water to which you add - for one eyebath – two drops of Tincture of Calendula or two drops of Tincture of Euphrasia (Eyebright), or both together. Two tablespoons of Rosewater, one of plain boiled water. Add a few drops of Tincture of Euphrasia.

See also Eyes

Constipation

Constipation is the result of the body's failure to expel its wastes swiftly and efficiently. They are thus retained in the bowel or rectum for days, even weeks, instead of passing smoothly through to be excreted. The cause is usually defective diet: it is estimated that in Western diets - full of refined carbohydrates, sugar, processed foods and chemical additives, and deficient in natural roughage in the form of fruit, vegetables or whole grains, food takes up to three weeks to pass through the system instead of the day or two common in 'primitive' people. It is hardly surprising, that possibly fifty per cent of the population in the affluent countries is constipated, and that many people are aggravating the problem by dosing themselves regularly with laxatives and purges which in the end discourage the muscles of the colon and bowel from functioning normally.

Since it's so common, constipation has attained music-hall joke status, but there's nothing very funny about what chronic constipation can do to the body, as the toxins generated by the wastes retained in your bowel are re-absorbed into – and circulated through - your bloodstream. Among the illnesses and complaints to which constipation may be a significant contributing factor are Arthritis, Rheumatism, gout, diverticulitis and appendicitis. It is increasingly suspected of preparing the perfect terrain for cancer, and among the many minor disorders to which it gives 'rise are fatigue, Headaches, Depression, Hypertension, Skin Problems and Catarrh.

The best remedy for most cases of constipation is true kitchen medicine -' a complete reform of diet, cutting out white bread, white flour, refined cereals, sugar, excess fat, too much tea, coffee and alcohol, and the substitution of a generous amount of fresh or dried fruit, vegetables rich in fibre such as cabbage, spinach, carrots, potatoes (eaten skin and all) and wholegrain cereals. Regular exercise is vital.

Mild forms of constipation will respond to this treatment which, as an emergency measure, you can supplement by a course of any of the mild herbal remedies for constipation listed below, or by including foods in your diet which as well as being nutritious offer an active solution to the problem.

Linseeds, for instance, are mucilaginous and highly absorbent: they will help create bulk in the rectum to aid the formation of softer, more easily passed stools.

Any of the following foods can be added regularly to your diet.

Soak a teaspoon of Linseeds in a cupful of hot water for two hours, drink the tea and eat the seeds with a spoon, adding a little lemon juice and honey if you like. Fink's Linusit Gold organically cultivated linseed which you can sprinkle over breakfast cereal, a tablespoonful a day, or eat with yogurt or milk, is available in most health food shops.

Psyllium Seeds work in much the same way as Linseeds. Put a couple of teaspoons of the little dark seeds in a cupful of warm water, and let it stand for five minutes while they swell into a gelatinous but completely tasteless goo. Taken in the morning, once during the day, and again at bedtime, it will help carry old faecal matter right out of the colon to give your system a thorough spring-clean.

Prunes are the classic nursery remedy - and highly effective.

Wash them thoroughly, then pour boiling water over them, and let soak overnight. Eat four or five with their' Juice for breakfast.

Herbal remedies to be taken occasionally, or for short courses
Yellow Dock root is tonic and cleansing as well as laxative.

Simmer 1 oz (25 g) of the root in 1 pint (550 rnl) of water for twenty minutes. Strain: drink a small cupful 3 times a day. Elder Flowers are another mild laxative, equally cleansing. Take a teaspoon infused for ten minutes in a cup of boiling water.

Senna is the classic laxative unless yours is the kind caused by tension or spasm of the bowel (producing intermittent bouts of mild diarrhoea) in which case it will make matters worse: for such cases, consult a practitioner. For ordinary constipation, try one of the excellent made-up formulae containing Senna.

Among the best of these are: Gerard House's Gladlax Natural Herb Tablets which contain Holy Thistle, Aloes, Fennel Powder, Myrrh Powder, Skullcap, Powdered Valerian, Powdered Lime Flowers; Potter's Natural Herb Tablets with Aloes, Cascara, Dandelion Root, Fennel, Holy Thistle, Myrrh, Senna Leaf and Valerian Root. These are both fairly typical formulae, the Aloes, Cascara and Senna operating as laxatives, the Fennel added to prevent 'griping' since they are quite powerful laxatives, the Dandelion for its tonic and cleansing properties, the Myrrh for its antiseptic qualities and the Lime, Skullcap and Valerian to calm the system after all this activity!

A course of Potter's Lion Cleansing Herbs could clear up an obstinate case of constipation: take it once a day for a week, and then give your system a rest. It comes in the form of a coarse powder, to be taken dry, washed down with a drink of water or tea. It contains Senna, for its stimulating laxative effect together with another laxative, Frangula Bark, with Fennel to counteract any possible irritant effect, bulk-producing Psyllium Seeds, Elder Flowers to help break up mucus and Mate as stimulant .

For acute or chronic constipation however – especially when it has persisted for years, you will need professional advice. A herbalist will not only advise on diet, but will prescribe herbs that can cleanse, tone and strengthen the entire system. Sudden, painful and persistent constipation, especially if there is no identifiable reason such as a radical change of diet or drinking water, may possibly indicate a blockage or other bowel disorder and a doctor should be consulted immediately.

See also Digestive Problems, Piles.

Convalescence

After an operation, or a long and serious illness, the tonic herbs can help to restore your strength and vitality, build up stamina, resistance and energy, and generally tone up the body.

The most highly reputed of all the tonics is Ginseng, which has remarkable powers to restore all the systems of the body to normal function after illness or surgery. Since it is a stimulant, it should not be used in combination with too many others - tea, coffee and alcohol in particular - so cut your intake of these to a minimum while you are taking Ginseng. And if you suffer from high blood pressure, don't take it at all.

Siberian Ginseng *(Eleutherococcus senticosus),* is milder, and can be taken when Ginseng would be over-stimulating. You could, therefore, start taking it much earlier in convalescence, with splendid results. It's also useful as an all-purpose tonic for when you're feeling generally listless, overworked, or below par. But don't expect instant results – it won't work as.a quick overnight pick-me-up. Like Ginseng, its best results come from a long course _. at least a fortnight.

One of the rare herbal remedies which have been submitted to the full range of modern efficacy and toxicity tests is Bio- Strath Elixir from Switzerland. It has also undergone a number of trials - in hospitals and elsewhere - and performed impressively in all of them, demonstrating a high level of usefulness in improving stamina, endurance, mental function, as well as assisting recovery from serious illness, surgery, or debilitating therapy such as X-ray treatment. It's also valuable for improving resistance generally: if my children start to look

pale and peaky, I put them on a course of it immediately. Bio-

Strath Elixir is made from plasmolysed *candida utilis* yeast cells, which are first fed on a number of health-giving herbs, including Angelica, Lemon Balm, Chamomile, Elder, Fennel, Lavender, Sage and Thyme, and then used to ferment a mixture of orange juice, malt and honey.

Floradix Formula is a real old-fashioned herbal tonic from Salus-Haus in Germany: it is rich in vitamins and minerals from herbs such as Nettles, Ocean Kelp, Spinach and Wheat germ, and from concentrates of fruit such as Red Grapes and Blackcurrants. The suggested daily dose provides 15 mg of absorbable iron - a shot in the arm for that run-down, washed-out feeling.

Fenugreek - a 'rejuvenator' in traditional medicine - is a superb tonic, rich in traces of B vitamins. It helps to cleanse your body of all the pockets of waste that may have piled up as mucus, thus aiding their digestion and elimination. A teaspoon of the seeds steeped for ten minutes in a cupful of boiling water can be taken three times a day.

Vervain is the first name that comes into a herbalist's mind when prescribing for that run-down, depressed state that can follow flu or other acute infectious illnesses. Take one ounce (30 g) of the dried herb, pour over it a pint (550 ml) of boiling water, steep for ten minutes, strain and drink a wineglassful, cold, three times a day. It is also available as a tea flavoured with orange.

Avens is another excellent post-flu treatment. In fact you can use it all the way through the illness, drinking it hot while you're flu-ridden since it is mildly diaphoretic and tonic, and then taking it cold to help you over the after-effects.

Slippery Elm is the perfect invalid food, toning and purifying the body as well as providing easily digested nutrients. Make gruel of it by adding hot water or milk, or both, sweeten it with a little honey, and add a dash of Cinnamon, Clove, Nutmeg and Ginger to improve the taste as well to give a fillip to a run-down digestive system. Bioforce Ginsavena is a pleasant way to take a ready-made tonic: in liquid form, to be added a few drops at a time to water or a tisane, it combines the nerve-strengthening, tonic properties of Ginseng and Oats.

The best-selling formula of Muir's in Edinburgh has for years been their Tonic Tablets, containing a range of stimulating, tonic, anti-depressive herbs, a lovely herbal pick me-up for anyone recovering from an operation, or a long debilitating illness. The tablets contain Agrimony, Kola, Goldenseal, Skullcap, Valerian Root, Motherwort, and Lime Flowers.

Corns

Corns are plugs of dead horny tissue, usually on the feet and caused by badly-fitted shoes. A chiropodist should deal with enlarged or painful corns, but minor cases can be dealt with in the following ways:

Tape on a slice of Lemon overnight, or paint with fresh Lemon Juice.

After soaking your feet in a hot footbath to which you have added Epsom Salts, paint the corn with Oil of Turpentine and cover it with lint or a plain sterile dressing.

Tape on a thin slice of Garlic overnight, or crush the juice of one clove on to the small square of gauze in the middle of a sticking plaster to apply to the corn.

See also Bunions, Feet, Verrucas.

Coughs

When the mucous membrane lining your throat or bronchial tract becomes inflamed and irritated, it produces extra mucus.

A cough is a reflex action of the body designed to dislodge and eject that mucus. So medicines aimed at suppressing the cough are no help at all. You need something to soothe and heal the inflamed mucous membrane to stop it producing this excess mucus, and something to make your cough more productive so that it gets rid of it fast - an 'expectorant', in fact. A good cough medicine will also deal with any virus or bacteria that have settled into the trouble spot and are multiplying.

It seems a lot to ask of any medicine, but there are plenty of safe, homely herbal remedies that can do one, two - or even all three. I've listed them under Bronchitis. A cough, incidentally, is a sign that the inflammation and infection of a head cold are starting to spread down into throat and lungs, so don't neglect it, or you could wind up with Bronchitis.

If a cough is persistent or painful, or if it brings up brown or discoloured mucus, or blood, consult a doctor.

See also Bronchitis, Colds, Influenza, Laryngitis, and Whooping Cough.

Cuts, grazes and scratches *see* Children's Ailments.

Cystitis

Inflammation and infection of the bladder should always be referred to a doctor as a matter of the utmost urgency, since infection can easily spread to the kidneys, and cause serious and lasting damage. Fever, agonising discomfort when urinating, persistent pain radiating upwards into the loins and lower back, and traces of blood in your urine are all indications of this worsening of the condition. Cystitis is most emphatically *not* a disease -for self-diagnosis. The herbal practitioner can call on a wide range of useful herbs in the treatment of cystitis: urinary disinfectants such as Bearberry and Buchu, as well as those that will soothe inflammation and promote healing, relax muscle spasm, and normalise the flow of urine. He would certainly also prescribe herbs for the general condition that has allowed such a serious infection to establish itself, and may advise a simple blood-cleansing diet.

If you have already consulted your family doctor, you may be taking medication - usually in the form of antibiotics – for the condition. However, conventional treatment is not invariably successful, nor does it always produce immediate relief. Indeed, it may very well make matters worse, since antibiotics slaughter intestinal flora indiscriminately, good guys and bad guys alike. You need the benign microbial flora to keep your gut functioning sweetly and efficiently – and control your cystitis. In order to repopulate your gut, take acidophilus capsules, and eat plenty of yogurt.

Meanwhile, here is a simple remedy which can be taken at the same time as any drugs your doctor may have ordered, to help soothe and heal the inflamed lining of the bladder.

Marshmallow Root is soothing, healing, and mildly diuretic: if you can get the powdered root, pour a cupful of boiling water onto a teaspoon of it, and stir well, letting it stand for 30 minutes. It will form into a glutinous paste, which can be sweetened with a very little honey. Take it three times a day, before meals. The dried, unpowdered root can either be grated, or chopped up into smaller pieces, and 1ounce (30 g) of it simmered in 1 pint (550 ml) of water for 30 minutes: take a cupful as above.

Potter's Antitis Tablets have given relief to many chronic sufferers. They contain urinary disinfectants and herbs with an astringent or antiseptic as well as a diuretic action, including Buchu, Bearberry, Horsetail and Shepherd's Purse.

Dandruff and other Hair Problems

Like any other part of your skin, your scalp is a clear indication of your general health: whoever saw someone seriously ill with lustrous healthy hair? Dandruff may be a mild form of dermatitis - step up your Vitamin B intake with lots of whole grains and wheat germ. Cut down on sugar or cut it out altogether if possible and you will probably see a steady improvement. Strong 'medicated' shampoos may make matters worse by irritating the scalp. Too frequent washing won't help either, nor will extra-hot water for the shampoo.

The best shampoos to use are mild, natural, soap free, containing herbs that will cleanse (and, if necessary, disinfect), and tone the scalp by stimulating its circulation - equally good for dry or 'greasy hair. Particularly good shampoos: Nettle Shampoo with Rosemary, or their cool, spicy Clove and Dandelion Shampoo.

The Body Shop sells an Orange Spice Shampoo containing the oils of stimulating and antiseptic spices – including; Thyme, Cassia, Cinnamon Leaf and Clove for itchy, scaling scalps, their Aromatherapy Scalp Oil blends Lavender,

Juniper, Rosemary and Cyprus oils: it should be massaged into the scalp and left on for half an hour before shampooing.

Culpeper's Rosemary Herbal Shampoo, a powder shampoo you make up yourself which also contains such traditional hair-conditioners as Southern wood, Balm and Quassia.

Weleda's Lemon and Melissa Shampoo, containing essential oils of Pine and Lemon.

Potter's Medicated Extract of Rosemary, containing Rose Geranium Oil, Rosemary Oil and Wintergreen with borax, in a spirit base, will cleanse and stimulate the scalp.

If you can't afford special shampoos, use a mild baby shampoo, using lukewarm water and giving your scalp plenty of massage, with a cold rinse afterwards.

Strong infusions of Thyme, Rosemary, Sage or Nettles will all help. After shampooing, rub them well into the hair and scalp, massage for a few minutes, and then rinse out.

And if you're going to wash your hair in the morning, massage a little Witch Hazel into it last thing at night.

Depression

Depression is a word covering a multitude of mental or emotional states, ranging all the way from a mild and passing gloom to a state of deep and settled unhappiness. Acute sufferers often seem to have withdrawn from life itself and need expert help, fast. In mild cases life itself with all its vicissitudes may be the cause. But if you feel dispirited and depressed there may well be a physical explanation. Vitamin or mineral deficiencies in your diet may be the cause. Depression may be due to a deficiency of zinc, and often responds to zinc supplementation with dramatic speed. See under Anorexia Nervosa for a simple, inexpensive way to find out if this could be so in your case. Vitamin B deficiencies can often have this effect, as, for instance, is common in some forms of Post-natal Depression. Some women on the Pill suffer a Vitamin B6 deficiency. Taking a supplement, and boosting your all-round intake of the B vitamins, can often solve this problem.

Changes in the fluid balance of your body can influence your emotional state - the weepy sensitivity that afflicts some women just before their period is linked with increased fluid retention. Many drugs have a depressant side effect – among them painkillers and some antibiotics, especially when taken in high doses, even tranquillisers. Depression is also a typical symptom of allergy, sometimes severe enough to take its victims into psychiatric care. Sufferers are susceptible to a wide range of substances, most of them man-made, such as the fumes' from gas, petrol or paint solvents, chemical food additives, and even quite common items in a normal diet such as tea, coffee or wheat. Illness, particularly liver complaints, often brings depression as an after-effect, when the body's reserves of strength and vitality have been seriously depleted post- flu depression is another classic case.

For all these various forms of depression, millions of pounds' worth of tranquillisers are prescribed annually. But almost anything that tranquillisers can do, herbs have for centuries done better, or at least as well, and they have the added merit of being safe and non-addictive medicines. They work by soothing away tensions, and nourishing, toning and strengthening the nervous system. Some of them supply nutrients 'essential to the healthy function of our nerves.

Skullcap, for instance, is rich in calcium, potassium and magnesium. Amazingly, some of the most effective are among the mildest: Chamomile, Lemon Balm and Catnip are all herbs you can safely give to children when they are feverish, upset or out of sorts, while Oats - real nerve-food - can be among the, first cereals a baby eats when it switches to solid food. Valerian, Lady's Slipper and Vervain are other gentle, effective tranquillisers.

If you suffer from severe or chronic depression, seek expert advice. For milder forms of depression, try one of the' following remedies:

Lemon Balm tea is a fine tonic for depression from whatever cause. Infuse one teaspoon, covered, in boiling water, for ten minutes. Or you can make up a day's supply, one ounce (30 g) to a pint (550 ml) of water. Take three times a day, the last dose at bedtime.

Oats are excellent for depression following an illness, since they're nourishing as well as tonic to the nerves. A herbalist will prescribe oats in tincture form. You can make a thin porridge of them, adding honey or raisins to sweeten it.

Vervain seems almost specifically designed for post-flu depression. Infuse one teaspoonful, or a teabag, covered in a cup of boiling water and drink three times a day.

Drink Chamomile tea, a few heads to a cupful of boiling water, or use a teabag.

Catnip is very soothing, so if you have any growing in your garden, add a couple of the leaves to infuse with your Chamomile tea.

Rosemary is high in calcium in an easily assimilated form, and is particularly good for that low, run-down feeling after illness.

Steep a teaspoonful, preferably fresh, in a clip of boiling water, and infuse, covered, for ten minutes. Sweeten with honey.

If you have a Lavender bush in your garden, add a pinch of the flowering tops to any of these infusions to enhance their tonic effect.

A particularly delightful remedy for depression is Lemon Leaf Tea, a fragrant spicy mix of all the lemony herbs including Verbena, Balm and Thyme, with Fennel. Serve hot or cold with a slice of Lemon.

For mild but chronic depression try Ginseng. See Convalescence for directions on how to take it.

See also Nerves, Post-natal Depression, Pre-menstrual Tension

Diarrhoea

Chronic diarrhoea needs expert diagnosis and treatment, as does sudden violent diarrhoea accompanied by sharp pain and fever. Diarrhoea may also be caused by a course of antibiotics, which slaughter the benign bugs that keep your gut functioning normally and sweetly the rest of the time. Eat yogurt to stave off the worst of the damage. Most of the time, though, diarrhoea is simply your body's natural defence system efficiently working to throw out toxic matter as fast as possible. The best herbal remedies assist this action while soothing local pain and inflammation.

Powdered Rhubarb Root: Enough to cover your thumbnail, taken three times a day with a little water.

Agrimony is tonic and astringent. Add a teaspoonful of the herb to a cup of boiling water, infuse for ten minutes and allow to cool. Drink a wineglassful every two hours.

The spice rack can provide your cure. Try a teaspoonful of

Cinnamon, simmered in water for twenty minutes with a little added honey. Would you believe that fiery red Cayenne Pepper could work, too? Add a teaspoonful to a wineglass of warm water, sweeten with honey and swallow.

Marshmallow Root: An ounce (30 g) simmered for twenty minutes in a pint (550 ml) of water, produces a thick mucilage, which can be sweetened with a little honey and spiced with a dash of Cinnamon to make it drinkable. It soothes and heals fast. Powdered Comfrey Root works the same way - add a teaspoonful to a cup of boiling water.

Add a few drops of essence of Peppermint to a cupful of hot water and sip it as hot as possible. Repeat every two to three hours.

Meadowsweet tea, made with a teaspoonful of the dried herb infused for ten minutes in a cupful of not-quite-boiling water, is also useful.

Grated apple sounds too simple to be true, but try it if you have nothing else to hand. If you have Oats, simmer them for at least half an hour to make a thin gruel, and take teaspoons of it, sweetened with honey and with a little Cinnamon added to it.'

Always drink plenty of water preferably bottled spring water.

See also Spanish Tummy

Digestive Problems

Indigestion, gas, heartburn, flatulence, colicky pains, 'acidity' and stomach pains are all emergency signals sent up by a disordered stomach. Too much rich food and drink, irregular meals, gobbling your food, bolting a lunchtime sandwich, and the kind of nervous tension that goes straight to your stomach are all possible causes. When the old-fashioned Nanny said 'Chew your food slowly' she knew a thing or two. The process of digestion actually starts in the mouth, where chemical substances in your saliva start breaking down and processing food. When you rush a meal, half of it probably skips this first stage in the digestive process - putting an extra workload on your poor stomach. Fatty foods are another burden. Since they slow down the digestive processes, your stomach goes into overtime, producing superfluous digestive juices, many of them acid, with resulting discomfort to you. Sucking antacid pills makes matters worse: their high alkaline content knocks out the acids but does nothing to aid digestion. And if you go on taking antacids, your stomach will simply step up its acid production in response, paving the way for tomorrow's gastric ulcer.

If you're a frequent sufferer from this kind of problem, your diet probably heeds checking. Cut out - or at least cut down on - white sugar, white bread and flour, fried foods, animal fats, excess alcohol. Step up your intake of salads, fresh fruit and vegetables, and make sure that you get plenty of dietary fibre.

Aim for calmer, less rushed mealtimes - and remember what Nanny said about chewing.

Another common cause is a food or drink Allergy – one woman I know spent weeks swallowing tranquillisers and undergoing hospital tests for her chronic stomach pains till a kind friend suggested that her enthusiastic consumption of coffee might be responsible. She dropped it for a week, and the pains went away. Tea is another culprit.

I know of several people whose digestive problems – even those of allergic origin - have disappeared with almost magical swiftness when they adopted the Hay Diet - a healthy system of eating which avoids the consumption of concentrated starch and protein at the same meal: no bread, rice or potatoes with meat, for instance, no cheese with your bread, and either fish or chips. For a full description of how and why it works, together with menus and recipes.

If none of this helps and odd pains persists - especially if they are severe - consult an herbal practitioner.

Most digestive problems, you might say, start in the kitchen, so it seems appropriate that you can lay your hands on most of the effective herbal remedies for them without moving out of there, particularly if you have a well-stocked spice rack. Almost all the herbs and spices familiarly used in cooking are natural aids to digestion, stimulating, toning, warming and soothing. Parsley, 'Sage, Rosemary and Thyme, Garlic and Onions, Marjoram and Mint, Rosemary, Cumin, Cayenne and Fennel will all help your stomach cope with even the richest festive food. And the housewife with a window-sill, of culinary herbs in pots and a spice rack stocked with fresh supplies of aromatic spices can do more for her family's digestions than a truckload of antacid pills.

Here are some very simple remedies.

For flatulence or nausea, a teaspoonful of Cinnamon simmered in milk with a little honey.

A pinch of grated Nutmeg, taken the same way.

The juice of half a Lemon taken in hot water.

A teaspoon of Marjoram steeped, covered, in a cupful of boiling water for ten minutes.

A teaspoon of grated Ginger Root simmered, covered, in a cupful of boiling water for ten minutes. A teaspoonful of fresh or dried Basil Leaves, steeped, covered, in a cupful of boiling water for ten minutes - or chew the fresh leaves.

Hot Peppermint tea: For belching and farting, all the warm tropical spices are helpful - Cinnamon, as above; a teaspoonful of crushed

Caraway seeds, steeped in a cupful of boiling water, covered for twenty minutes. Half a dozen Cardamom pods, simmered, covered, in a cupful of water, with a sprinkle of grated Ginger or Nutmeg. (Always buy these fragrant spices in whole rather than ground form, and grate or grind them yourself. They'll preserve their aroma - and their medicinal value – much longer.) A teaspoonful of crushed Fennel Seeds, steeped for twenty minutes, covered, in a cupful of boiling water. A sprig of fresh Thyme, or a teaspoonful of dried Thyme, steeped, covered, in a cupful of boiling water for ten minutes.

For cramps and colicky pains, hot Peppermint tea - use a teabag. Hot Lemon Balm - use a teabag or better still, if you grow it, five or six fresh leaves steeped, covered, in a cupful of boiling water for ten minutes.

Hot Chamomile tea. Chamomile, Peppermint and Lemon Balm can be mixed if you prefer, and a dash of grated Ginger Root makes them even more effective.

Slippery Elm is a wonderful friend to the disordered stomach, soothing the irritated lining of the digestive tract: it's often combined with warming spices to stimulate and tone, alongside its demulcent activity. Take a teaspoonful of the powder, make it into a paste with cold water, pour on a cupful of boiling water, stirring all the time. Spice with a little Cinnamon, and sweeten with honey. Slippery Elm Tablets, which also contain. Cinnamon, Clove and Peppermint Oils.

Napier's Indigestion Tablets tackle the problem from several herbal angles: they contain Ginger, both warming and grateful to an upset stomach, Goldenseal, tonic and healing, Valerian for a calming effect, Myrrh to cleanse and disinfect, and Rhubarb and Dandelion to help elimination.

For acidity, Meadowsweet, that charming wild flower with the little creamy-white feathery cones, is invaluable. Steep an ounce of the herb in a pint of not-quite-boiling water, covered for ten minutes. It tastes quite pleasant, too. It contains a good dose of Meadowsweet - together With Medicinal Vegetable Charcoal to help absorb toxic wastes, a dash of Rhubarb to speed them on their way, and some of the digestive spices':" Anise, Caraway, Cardamom and Cinnamon.

If your digestive problems are the result of stress and strain, see under Nerves and Nervous Tension to help you to correct the underlying cause, and treat your symptoms as above.

See also Bad Breath, Colic, Constipation, Diarrhoea, Hiccoughs, Spanish Tummy, Travel Sickness, Ulcers.

Earache

Earache is one ailment that calls for instant action: untreated, a mild ache can develop into agonising pain, and the inflammation can lead to deafness or brain damage, so professional advice should be sought at the earliest possible moment. It often follows a Cold, a chill or an infectious disease like Measles, when the body's defences are run down.

It's also, I've noticed, quite common among children on holiday getting an earful of the polluted Mediterranean. Away from home and one's own family doctor, this can be particularly alarming, which is why I never travel without the simplest and most effective remedy - Garlic oil in capsule form, and a small ear dropper. Here's how to administer it.

Scrub your hands clean, and assemble Garlic oil capsule, ear dropper, needle, boiling water, sterile cotton wool, and teaspoon.

Heat the teaspoon in the boiling water+ warmth is immensely soothing to an aching ear - dip the needle into the water and pierce the capsule, squeeze it into the heated and dried teaspoon, and let it warm up a little. Draw it up into the dropper - test on the back of your hand that it's not too hot then gently drop two or three drops into the aching ear, plugging it gently afterwards with cotton wool. If you have no dropper, simply squeeze two or three drops straight onto the cotton wool and plug the ear with it.

Ear drops should *not* be used if you suspect that the ear drum may be perforated. Instead, simply put the Garlic oil,

Mullein oil or Lemon juice on a piece of sterile warmed cotton wool, tuck it first inside the ear and keep in place with a scarf.

Lemon juice is a powerful bactericide - squeeze a few drops of the juice on to a piece of warmed cotton wool and plug the ear with it.

Mullein oil is another traditional and reliable remedy for earache, which you can get by special order from Nelson's.

Compresses as hot as can be borne, on and around the ear, will greatly allay pain.

Eczema

Stress and fatigue are common causes of eczema, that itchy, scaling skin complaint. So are Allergies, the commonest of which, in this case, is to dairy products. A typical case is the bottlefed baby whose immature digestive system cannot cope with cow's milk. Infantile eczema is extremely rare in breastfed babies. If stress is the probable cause of your eczema, see under Nerves and Nervous Tension for suggested remedies.

If you suspect an allergy, start by eliminating *all* dairy foods from your diet for a week - milk, butter, cheese, yogurt. If your eczema is visibly improved, stay off them. Many allergies may clear up after the body is restored to its full healthy function, and after a prolonged rest from the offending allergen. For general treatment, see under Skin Problems

One of the most hopeful new treatments for eczema is the oil of a little plant called the Evening Primrose. Pioneering research on it was done in the 1960s by John Williams, of Bio- Oil Research, and numbers of clinical studies of Evening Primrose Oil have been set up by Efamol Ltd, as a result of which medical interest in this humble little yellow-flowered plant has grown steadily over the last decade. Its importance is that apart from human breast-milk, it is one of the only two known sources (the other is the blue-flowered Borage plant) of an essential fatty acid called gamma-linolenic acid (GLA for short). GLA is the precursor in our bodies of a vital series of prostaglandins, the tiny little regulators of cell activity throughout our bodies, and when we are healthy; our bodies make their own supplies of GLA from the cis-linoleic acid supplied in natural plant oils. But the process can be blocked by a number of factors - among them the wrong kind of fats, found in the hydrogenated oils used in food processing and many margarines; viral infections; a high intake of alcohol; zinc deficiency; aging; and radiation. Evening Primrose Oil skips the conversion stage to supply ready-made GLA, and

Eczema is just one of the conditions in which clinical study sponsored by Efamol has shown it to be effective in many cases. (See also under Premenstrual Tension, Hyperactivity in Children, Hangovers.) In this study, fairly high doses were taken by patients for twelve weeks; the dosage suggested by Efamol is eight to twelve 500 mg capsules a day, together with two tablets, taken twice a day, of Efavite, containing zinc, vitamins B3, B6 and C, which aid its absorption. Efamol also now supply the oil in tiny 10 ml dropper bottles, to be applied directly to the rough scaly patches of eczema.

Red Clover Flowers, bright orange Marigold Flowers and the tiny violet flowers and leaves of Hearr's-ease are among the attractive plants that herbalists particularly value in the treatment of eczema. You can make up an infusion of anyone of these, adding a teaspoon of the dried herb - or rather more of the fresh - to a cupful of boiling water for ten minutes. Strain, and drink three times a day.

Stinging Nettles - much less attractive - are equally effective. You can now buy Nettle teabags, or harvest your own. (Wear gloves, of course, and pick the young tops only from a spot where they are not contaminated by drifting pesticide or lead pollution from passing cars.) Make them into a tea by infusing a dessertspoonful to a cup of boiling water, for ten minutes.

Both Nettles and Heart's-ease figure in Weleda's Eczema Tea, which also contains Chamomile Flowers, Elder Flowers and Juniper-Leaf tips. Infuse a teaspoonful for 10 minutes in a cup of boiling water, covered.

Red Clover, Chaparral and Ginseng Tablets from Gerard House will help.

For external application, Burdock Leaves, Comfrey Leaves, Elder Flowers .or Chamomile Flowers can all be infused, covered. Add a handful to a pint of boiling water and steep for ten minutes. The strained infusion is cooled and used for soothing, disinfectant compresses. Comfrey is particularly helpful for flaking, scaling skin.

See also Skin Problems

Flatulence see under Digestive Problems

Eyes: Sore, Red or Inflamed

See under Conjunctivitis. Any of the eye-washes will help. If your blurry tired eyes are simply the result of lack of sleep, too much strain, too much alcohol (disastrous for bright eyes), atmospheric pollution - especially from cigarette smoke, or hangover - a used teabag applied as a cold compress, is fast and effective relief. A perfectly ordinary teabag will do, once used: if you need to cool it fast, put it in a small dish in the freezer compartment of your fridge for a couple of minutes.

Better still are Fennel or Chamomile teabags. And if you have Raspberry Leaf tea in the house, make some, strain, cool, and use as a cold compress.

Feet: Sore and Aching

Dancers, shop-assistants, policemen and women, traffic wardens, are among those likely to suffer from their feet at one time or another. Balto Foot Balm - which you can buy in small tubes or big jars, contains soothing, healing aromatic oils - Pine, Menthol, Eucalyptus, Camphor, with tonic seaweed - Bladderwrack - in an antiseptic, non-greasy base.

Weleda Foot Balm is made from soothing and astringent plant oils, including Rosemary, Lavender, Sage, Lemon and Geranium in a cooling, non-greasy base.

See also Athlete's Foot, Bunions, Corns, Verrucas.

Fevers

A slight fever and feeling of mild discomfort is often the first sign of an infection, and if the temperature rises steeply, obviously a doctor should be called. But the fever that accompanies a particularly nasty cold, or a bout of 'flu, is not itself an ailment, merely' an indication that your body's efficient defence mechanisms are making a bonfire of toxic wastes in your system. Such wastes are normally efficiently expelled through the bladder, rectum, skin and lungs. In an emergency, fever speeds up elimination through the skin by raising body heat to cause perspiration or even heavy sweating.

Treatment should not suppress the fever (though if it is high it must be controlled), but should gently assist the process of elimination.

Sudden high fevers - particularly in a child - are another matter altogether. Call the doctor without delay. Meanwhile, put the patient to bed in a well-ventilated room. If he or she is particularly hot and distressed, sponge down the body very gently with tepid water, covering up each limb immediately afterwards, and give plenty of liquids to drink, such as hot water with honey and the juice of a fresh Lemon.

For milder fevers, or fevers in their early stages, any of the following remedies are helpful:

Hot Peppermint tea. Use fresh leaves if you have them – a teaspoonful steeped, covered, for ten minutes in a cupful of boiling water. Alternatively, use a teabag.

Hot Yarrow tea. This is especially good for the early stages of Colds and Influenza: a teaspoonful of the dried herb steeped for ten minutes in a cupful of boiling water can be sweetened with honey.

Hot Elder Flower tea. Steep a teaspoonful of the dried blossoms in a cupful of boiling water. Add honey to taste.

Catnip tea. Steep a teaspoonful, covered, in a cupful of not quite- boiling water.

Hibiscus tea. Use a teabag and add plenty of lemon juice.

Lemon Balm. This is much the most pleasant to take of all the herbs for fever. If you can make it with fresh leaves from your own garden or window box, so much the better. A heaped teaspoonful of Yarrow, Elder Flower and Peppermint are often combined in a classic fever remedy. One ounce each of Elder Flowers and Peppermint and half an ounce of Yarrow are steeped, covered, in a pint of boiling water. When strained, keep warm and covered; drink a wineglass from time to time.

All of these herbs are taken hot to promote perspiration. Once the fever has subsided and you are on the road to recovery, you can continue the herb tea of your choice, but drink it cold, when its tonic and diuretic qualities will help to restore your appetite and shake off the depression that sometimes descends after a feverish illness.

Gums ; Sore, Spongy, Infected, Bleeding

Blood on your toothbrush? Don't ignore the sign ... the advertisement used to say. Infected, bleeding gums are a septic focus - a continual source of toxins that your body can well do without. See your dentist and check the obvious things. Are you brushing your teeth properly - and using floss or Interdens regularly? Not pushing a hard, damaging brush smack up against the gums all round? Nor are you, on the other hand, simply running a broken-down soft brush around, which never stimulates them or cleans out the crevices in between? Often good oral hygiene alone will clear-up long standing cases of gingivitis, and if your dentist doesn't nag at you to keep it up - find yourself a new dentist. Are you deficient in Vitamin C? A very common reason. Or in the B vitamins? Take extra wheat germ, liver, brewers' yeast and see if they help. The problem still with you? Check your calcium intake - take bone meal or dolomite tablets supplying up to 1000 mg daily for a fortnight at least, to see if it makes a difference. Meanwhile, take a two-week course of Echinacea - the best natural antibiotic - to clear lurking infection, and try anyone of the following to help disinfect, tone, firm and strengthen your gums. Just one treatment won't help: work at it night and morning for at least a week. Other remedies are:

Hot Red Sage tea. This is the common-or-garden Sage, which you may have on your kitchen windowsill. If not, you can buy it dried from suppliers of medicinal herbs. Take a teaspoonful of the dried herb (more of the fresh leaves) and steep, covered, in a cupful of boiling water for ten minutes. Strain. Use it as a mouthwash, swishing it in and around your teeth, and holding it in your mouth for as long as possible.

Thyme tea. This is made and used the same way.

Hot Lemon and water. Squeeze the juice of a Lemon into half a cup of hot water. Use the same way. Rinse out your mouth afterwards, or the acid may damage the enamel. It's a change from Sage or Thyme, but don't use Lemon this way more than once or twice a week.

Tincture of Myrrh. Buy it from the chemist. Put five or six drops in a small glass of warm water and use as above. Weleda's Gargle and Mouthwash is gum-firming and refreshing with its spicy mix of soothing, disinfecting, astringent plants and plant oils - Krameria Root, Myrrh, Sage, Geranium, Lavender, Eucalyptus and Peppermint among other things. Use a few drops of it in warm water for a mouthwash, or neat on a cotton-wool bud for direct application to the gums.

It's also useful for the sores caused by ill-fitting dentures, as is Tincture of Calendula. Apply it neat on cotton wool and an orange stick, or a cotton-wool bud.

Bio-Strath Chamomile formula combines the healing and bactericidal action of Chamomile with marvellously antiseptic Sage. Take ten to twenty drops in a little water every two hours to clear up a severe case. Use it first as a mouthwash, swilling it around your teeth, then swallow.

If you have problem gums, you can do without the potentially irritating detergents present in most ordinary toothpastes, which are readily absorbed through the mucous membranes of the mouth. The herbalist David Simpson suggests making up your own: take four parts of ordinary bicarbonate of soda to one part of powdered fennel seeds and one part of dolomite tablets, also ground to a powder.

A ready-made toothpaste recommended by several herbal practitioners is Parodontax, made by Madaus of Germany, which contains oils or tinctures of several healing and antiseptic plants, among them Myrrh, Krameria, Chamomile, Sage and Peppermint, in a sodium bicarbonate base. Weleda make several excellent toothpastes, including their Herbal one.

And my children love atoothpaste called Homeodent, made by the French homoeopathic company Boiron and available at Neal's Yard Apothecary. Formulated to counter pyorrhoea and gingivitis, it has a delicious liquoricey taste and contains healing, cleansing herbs - Plantain, Pokeroot, Horseradish, Marigold and Witch Hazel.

See also Toothache, Bad Breath

Haemorrhoids *see under* Piles.

Hangovers

If it's the worst ever and you want to die, you may have been drinking cheap plonk laced with dubious chemicals (see under Diarrhoea). Sleep, a darkened room, and the slow passage of time are your best hope. Meanwhile, sipping warm water with a little Lemon juice squeezed into it from time to time will probably be as helpful as anything.

Your head gets the ache, but it's actually your overworked liver that's complaining. A glass of hot water with a juice of Lemon squeezed into it, or a cup of hot Peppermint tea should help, particularly if you can lie down for half an hour afterwards. Any of the essential oils mentioned above may also help. And for the kind of racking morning-after head that makes you seriously consider signing the Pledge, Thornham Herbs China Light Tisane combines Rosemary, Lime Flowers, Peppermint, Hops and Lavender with a little Peppermint oil. Use a heaped teaspoon in a cup, fill with boiling water, cover, steep for ten minutes, and sip hot.

A herbal remedy to counter the hangover syndrome at several levels is Potter's new Herbprin - a sort of plant aspirin, as its name suggests: it contains Yarrow and Elder Flowers to help your system throw off the accumulated toxicity that is making you feel so dire. Poplar Bark and and White Willow Bark to soothe throbbing, inflamed blood-vessels, Cinnamon to soothe your stomach, and Cinchona and Capsicum for their tonic powers.

Essential fatty acid deficiency, caused by all that alcohol, may be the explanation of much hangover misery. Here too, it may be Evening Primrose Oil to the rescue. (See Eczema.)

Recent research suggests that half a dozen 500 mg Efamol capsules swallowed after too much booze can, make the following dawn seem a good deal brighter.

See also Headaches

Hay Fever

Hay fever is the result of the mucous membranes which line the nose and sinus passages becoming inflamed and irritated by contact with an allergen - typically, grass pollen. The membrane may be acutely sensitive either because of poor general health, or of stress. The condition may have been triggered originally by a food allergy, often to milk (see Allergies). If so, eliminating this or other allergens from the diet will improve general resistance, and diminish the severity of hay fever attacks accordingly. A supplement of Vitamin C and the full range of B vitamins, particularly pantothenic acid, often work wonders. Eating plenty of Garlic, Onions and Chives also helps.

Inflammation and irritation of mucous membrane, which produce the non-stop sneezing, the streaming reddened eyes, and - naturally - the edgy, irritable state of mind can be relieved and soothed by any of the aromatic herbs useful for asthmatic conditions (see Asthma). Particularly good are Thyme, Marjoram, Hyssop, Lavender, infused, covered, and drunk warm, with a little honey.

Hot Mullein tea, two teaspoons to a cupful of boiling water, will help to clear accumulated mucus. If you grow this attractive plant with its downy grey leaves (one of its country names is Velvet Plant) you should use the yellow flowers and the tea should stand until it is bright yellow.

Eyebright is a particularly useful herb for hay fever since it not only helps to clear accumulated mucus and reduce the irritable sensitivity of this tissue, but also to reduce inflammation in and around the eyes - particularly susceptible during hay-fever attacks. Infuse a heaped teaspoonful of the herb in a cupful of boiling water and drink it hot or cold three times a day during the hay-fever season.

Pure Lemon juice sniffed very gently up the nostrils will also cool and soothe, although the initial disagreeable sensation may come as rather a shock, and it will reduce the risk of getting a nasty head cold while your defences are down.

Alternatively, soak plugs of cotton wool in Lemon juice and push them gently into the nose.

Keep a bottle of Witch-Hazel-in the refrigerator during the hay-fever season. Use it for cold compresses for reddened and inflamed eyes.

Headaches

Headaches are probably the most common of all the minor ailments. Indigestion, eye strain, tiredness, grief, tension, liver upsets, menstrual problems, high blood pressure, low blood sugar - or just an unconscious need for attention, and sympathy - can all trigger that familiar unpleasant throbbing around the temples. So can a past injury that caused concussion or jarring of the spine. Some drugs have headaches as a side effect - the Pill has been associated with cases of migraine, and migraine itself, the worst of all headaches, can have several contributory causes. An Allergy to certain chemicals or foods can give you a headache. Hangover headaches can be the worst of the lot.

Professional herbalists dislike ·treating symptoms on their own: they prefer to get at the root of the problem. Those with a blinding headache may feel less purist about the matter. If so, they could try Potter's new Herbprin, designed chiefly to allay the throbbing, aching pain of a headache, no matter how it all began. For its formula, see under Hangovers.

The tension headache

Any of the simple remedies for Nervous Tension will help ease this kind of headache, when the blood vessels in the head are swollen and inflamed, and the neck muscles tensed.

Lavender is among the most effective. Make an infusion of two teaspoons of the flowering tops in a cupful of boiling water, steep, covered, for ten minutes. Alternatively rub two or three drops of the Essential Oil of Lavender into your temples, or put two or three drops of the oil on a lump of sugar and eat it. Lime Flower tea will help relax the blood vessels in the head. To make it even more effective, drink it with your feet in the hottest footbath you can stand, and an icy cloth applied to the nape of your neck. Stimulating essential oils, applied to the forehead can often relieve this kind of headache.

Try Peppermint, Rosemary, Wintergreen, Olbas Oil, Tiger Balm, if you happen to have any of them in the house. Rub a few drops into the temples.

Early morning headaches

The kind you wake up with. If you keep on getting them, you may have low blood sugar, caused by a high intake of refined carbohydrates and sugar. Fatigue and lack of sleep can give you the same dull ache: the best thing I know is a hot infusion of

Skullcap, a teaspoon to a cup, infused covered in boiling water for ten minutes. Lime Flowers will also help. So will Dandelion Root tea, made by simmering an ounce (30 g) of the sliced roots in a pint (550 ml) of water for fifteen minutes.

Drink a wineglassful at a time.

Headaches due to digestive or elimination problems

These can also be cleared by Dandelion tea, which tackles the problem energetically at source, toning up and stimulating the liver. Any of the Hangover remedies will also help with this brand of headache. So will an infusion of Rosemary: a teaspoon steeped covered for 10 minutes in a cupful of boiling water; leave it to cool, and drink half a cupful at a time.

Headaches associated with menstruation

See under Menstrual Problems.

Migraine headaches

See under Migraine

Hepatitis, Jaundice, and other Liver Problems

Any illness affecting the liver and gall-bladder needs professional attention: get medical advice. People with serious liver problems usually feel much too ill to eat, but should be encouraged to drink plenty of bottled spring water, with the juice of half a Lemon freshly squeezed into each glass. Lemon is not only rich in minerals the body needs - potassium, calcium, phosphorus and magnesium, as well as Vitamin C, but it's cleansing and mildly stimulating to the jaded liver.

Elder Flower tea, Chamomile and Fennel are also good for the liver, so they make good sickroom drinks for jaundice cases.

When the worst is over and you can face food again, keep fats to a minimum, but eat plenty of fresh vegetables, especially Radishes, Beetroot, Chicory, Fennel, Celery and Artichoke, according to season - all are particularly good for the liver. The king of all the liver tonics is Dandelion. Use the leaf at first, infusing a teaspoonful in a cup of boiling water for ten minutes and drink three times a day. After a week or two, when life is back to normal, make a tea from the root - a much stronger tonic. Simmer a teaspoonful of the root in a cupful of water for twenty minutes and drink three times daily. Do not sweeten. Dandelion is rich in easily assimilated minerals. You can also add young Dandelion leaves to your salads, if they happen to be in season. And even if you feel that life without tea or coffee is hardly worth living, try switching for a while to Dandelion coffee, to give your liver a breather. There are various brands on the market, including one mixed with Chicory, or you can buy packets of the roasted root, and either simmer them for ten minutes and drink the resulting coffee coloured brew, or else grind them and use like instant coffee.

Strengthening tonics are necessary to aid the body's full recovery from the devastating effects of liver problems on its efficient functioning (see Convalescence). A particularly good one is Bio-Strath's Artichoke Formula, in which an extract of this plant is combined with extract of Thistle Seeds - both of them proved in scientific trials to stimulate the flow of bile by more than fifty per cent - and Peppermint, with its soothing properties.

Hiccoughs

Nobody is absolutely sure what produces this spasmodic stricture of the diaphragm. Muscular or nervous tension could be one explanation, local irritation another. Try any of the following:

A teaspoonful of freshly squeezed Lemon juice.

The juice of half an Orange.

Teaspoonful doses of Onion juice - grate it finely, then crush it through a wire sieve, if you don't have a Garlic press.

Chew a leaf of fresh Tarragon or Mint, if you have either.

If you have Gripe-Water for a baby in the house, take some of that;

15 of Potter's Antispasmodic Drops in a little water.

A couple of Vegetable Charcoal Tablets swallowed with half a glass of water, and a couple of Neurelax Tablets, or any other herbal formulation containing Valerian: see under Nerves and Nervous Tension.

(There are, of course, any number of 'mechanical' hiccoughs cures, of which the most reliable seem to be drinking from the opposite side of a glass, and, even better, stretching your arms high above your head while someone gives you sips of water. If you are alone on a desert island, the same effect can be achieved by bracing the inside of one forearm across the back of your head as hard as you can, and drinking sips of cold water from a glass held in your free hand. It sounds complicated, but rarely fails.)

Influenza

Some people rather like getting mild flu. They see it as a perfect excuse for spending two days in bed, away from office, shopping or school, waited on hand and foot - with any luck and rather enjoying the rest. For these mild cases, treat as for Fevers.

For the much nastier, more serious flu that brings aching heads and bones, and a general wrung-out feeling, there's a herb which seems designed as a specific remedy - learned by desperate white settlers in New England from Indian herbals, and christened Boneset because it coped with a highly unpleasant form of flu called Break-bone Fever. You can buy it in dried form from herbal suppliers -lay in a packet at the start of winter. Infuse ½ ounce (15 g) of it in 1 pint (550 ml) of boiling water for fifteen minutes, then give it hot, a small wineglassful at a time, every hour or so until the patient is perspiring, then slowly taper off the doses.

Even after quite mild cases of flu, people often feel unexpectedly run-down or low in spirits. See Convalescence for a good herbal pick-me-up and Depression for how to beat the post-flu blues.

Prevention

When there's flu about, an old Victorian remedy, Life Drops, could help keep it - or colds - at bay. Muir's Life Drops contain Capsicum and Peppermint Oil to keep your circulation in fine fettle, and Elder Flowers and Yarrow to keep your eliminative system in good order with their diaphoretic, warming action - particularly valuable in winter.

Take a few drops when you've got chilled through to the bone, too. Mr Low of Muir's tells me that he takes 5 drops in a little water, night or morning, every day in winter - and that he hasn't had a cold in twenty years.

See also Convalescence, Depression, Fevers

Insect Bites and Stings

Some people are abnormally sensitive to insect bites and stings, which may cause a reaction so severe as to need urgent medical attention. In these rare cases treat for shock immediately and get to a doctor as quickly as possible (see under Shock). Bee stings and ant stings are both acid: immersing the stung bit of the victim in ice-cold water to which you've added baking soda will help. Remember to pull or scrape out the bee sting.

Wasp stings, just to be different, are alkaline: vinegar will therefore help. These remedies are useful for insect bites and stings:

Pure Lemon juice, or grated Lemon rind with all the oils in it.

A compress of grated Onion - or a slice of Onion.

A compress of ice-cold Witch Hazel. Keep a bottle in the refrigerator while on holiday.

Oil of Eucalyptus, applied neat.

The essential oil of Lavender, applied neat.

Nelson's Pyrethrum Liquid is made of tinctures prepared from several useful plants, among them Calendula, Arnica, the friendly Dock that soothes nettle stings, pain-killing St john's Wort, Echinacea to guard against blood-poisoning, Labrador Tea

- used in Greenland to soothe itches and irritation – and Pyrethrum itself, or Persian Pellitory. Pyrethrum Liquid can be used as repellent - or as remedy. Dab it on neat if it's the remedy you want.

Nelson's Urtica Urens Ointment is made from the Stinging Nettle and used in true homoeopathic style to counteract the pain they cause.

To soothe the irritation and inflammation remaining after the worst of the pain has subsided use cold compresses of Tincture of Calendula, or Calendula Ointment.

Prevention

Have you ever wondered why the mosquitoes always seem to go for the tourists, while leaving the natives strictly alone? A very likely explanation is that they are repelled by the smell of Garlic - however faint - that assails keen insect nostrils from the skins of those who eat a lot of it. So eat a lot of it - and the same goes for Thyme, Lemon, Onion, Marjoram and Basil.

They don't much care for Lavender, either, so sprinkle Lavender Water around your bed at night, or put a couple of drops of essential oil of Lavender on the pillow. Cut 3J1 Onion in half and put it by your bed, unless it repels you too, in which case leave it on the windowsill. In the case of severe bites, rub a cut Onion over exposed limbs, or make a solution of Nelson's

Pyrethrum Liquid and sponge over exposed areas.

Insomnia
There are dozens of herbs that will help to soothe the frayed, jangling nerves, the edginess and tension, the weariness of brain or muscle or the anxiety that can mean nights of sleepless

tossing and turning. None of them is truly addictive, in the strict sense of the word, but no remedy that acts upon the central nervous system should be taken for weeks on end, night after night. If you become psychologically dependent upon any remedy, however safe or harmless, for your night's sleep, your insomnia problems remain unsolved. If they arise from tension and strain, see under Nerves. If you feel tired, run-down, see under Convalescence and give yourself a course of tonic herbs if you can't take a break. If the problem could be digestive, see under Digestive Problems. If none of this works, a herbal practitioner could make more effective suggestions, based on your personal history. For occasional insomnia, here are some simple remedies to try:

Chamomile tea: Infuse, covered, in a cupful of boiling water, or use a teabag.

Catnip tea: Infuse a teaspoonful of the herb, covered, in a cupful of near-boiling water for ten minutes. Very tranquillising.

Hops are a reliable old country remedy for insomnia: try a teaspoon of their papery heads, infused for ten minutes in a cupful of boiling water, sweetened with honey. To double the dose, try sleeping on a Hop pillow - Culpeper and some gift shops sell them. There is a bath oil based on Hops for a calming bed-time bath.

Lime tea: A teaspoon of Lime Flowers infused in a cupful of boiling water is also effective in calming restless, nervous states of mind.

The French herbalist Maurice Messegue recalls being put in a bath of Lime Flowers and Leaves as a child when he couldn't sleep - with magical results. You could follow suit with any of the herbs I've mentioned. Make an extra-strong infusion, strain and pour it into a warm bedtime bath, then drink an ordinary infusion of the same herb once in bed. Bedtime baths should be warm rather than hot. For a marked tranquillising effect, add two or three drops of the essential oil of Marjoram or Lavender on the surface, and swish it around with your hand. Laze in it for ten minutes, eyes closed, and then take yourself peacefully to bed.

Passionflower doesn't sound as though it ought to be good for promoting sweet sleep, but it's one of the finest remedies for insomnia. Potter's make Passionflower tablets – called Passiflora, the botanic name of the herb. Take at bedtime, washed down with one of the soothing herbal tisanes already mentioned.

Bridal Orange Blossom oughtn't to be good for sound sleep either, you'd think, but it is, in fact, highly soporific in infusions, and has sometimes brought relief where even powerful drugs have failed. You can buy Orange Blossom teabags.

Weleda's Avena Sativa Compound is mild, safe and relaxing, combining the sedative action of Passionflower, Valerian and Hops with the nerve-restoring action of Oats.

There are several delicious bedtime herbal blended teas now available, in which these and other calming, sleep-inducing herbs are used. Celestial Seasonings' Sleepy time Tea contains Chamomile, Passionflower, Orange Blossom and Lime Flowers among other good things; Jill Davies's 'Evening Peace' has Elderflower, Wood Betony, Chamomile and Hops;

Heath & Heather's Night Time Tea is another soporific blend.

Laryngitis

A dry itchy throat, an irritating cough, can be symptoms of an inflamed larynx which could leave you literally speechless.

Laryngitis usually follows a cold, and may be accompanied by fever. Any of the remedies for Sore Throat will help it – see that section. Sage or Thyme tea, used as a gargle and drunk afterwards in small doses is particularly effective. '

Weleda's Gargle & Mouth Wash is useful. Take a teaspoonful in a glass of warm water, gargle repeatedly, but do not drink it afterwards.

A few drops of Olbas Oil rubbed into the throat will also help to counter infection.

See also Cold, Coughs, Fevers, Sore Throat

Menstrual Problems

Seek expert advice for serious problems associated with the menstrual cycle, or the menopause. As well as giving individual advice on diet, herbalists can draw on a wide range of herbs that long experience or recent research has shown to be valuable, some with names that are eloquent of their use - Squaw Weed, Cramp Bark, Motherwort. A healthy diet, plenty of fresh air and exercise, and an adequate intake of vitamins and minerals are all important. Supplements of Vitamin B6, for instance, have cleared up long-standing menstrual problems for thousands. of women. If you've ruled out these deficiencies, try the following simple remedies.

If they don't work, consult a qualified practitioner.

Pre-Menstrual Tension, Headache, Depression, breast discomfort and fluid retention are symptoms experienced with varying degrees of severity, in the days immediately preceding their period. For many, P.M.T. is a regular prostrating ordeal. In a study at St Thomas's Hospital in London, 65 women suffering from P.M.T. were treated with Efamol Oil of Evening Primrose (see Eczema), after they had failed to respond to Vitamin B6 or hormone treatment. Only 15% said they felt no better and 61% reported that *all* their symptoms were eased. The dosage is around two 500 Efarnol capsules with one Efavite morning and evening: you may need less or more. The Pre-Menstrual Tension Advisory Service, recently set up in this country, has successfully counselled hundreds of women on nutritional and non-drug answers to this problem:

American research which they draw on suggests that deficiencies of magnesium as well as B6 - the two work closely together - may be responsible: good dietary sources of magnesium are soy beans, cashew nuts, almonds, peanuts, whole-wheat flour, brown rice and green vegetables - all part of any healthy diet.

For the dull headache that often accompanies a period, try Motherwort tea. Infuse one ounce (30 g) in a pint (550 ml) of boiling water, or a teaspoon to a teacup for ten minutes. Drink a wineglassful at a time after meals. Chamomile is also useful teabag can be used - but not if the periods are heavy.

For cramps and a feeling of heaviness, Raspberry Leaf tea is a favourite remedy. Infuse a teaspoonful in a cupful of boiling water for ten minutes. Drink hot three times a day for the two or three days before your period, or take half an ounce of Chamomile, infuse it in a pint. of boiling water, strain and add the tea to half an ounce of Cramp Bark with a pinch of powdered Ginger Root. Simmer for ten minutes. Drink a small glassful three times a day. You can also use this as a very comforting hot fomentation over the womb.

Gerard House make a Cramp Bark Tablet, which can be taken with a cup of Chamomile tea, or simply with water.

For painful periods which may be associated with a Digestive Problem. Potter's Uterine Sedative Tablets contain Bearberry and Gentian, both tonic to the stomach, and Motherwort, Valerian, Pulsatilla and Vervain for their relaxing, sedative effect.

For the fluid retention that often produces that heavy, bloated feeling in a period (it's also, incidentally, a fairly common side effect of the Pill) Dandelion tea is the best and safest diuretic. Infuse a teaspoon of the leaves in a cupful of boiling water for ten minutes and drink hot three times a day, after meals.

To check excessive bleeding, an infusion of Yarrow: a teaspoon of the dried herb steeped covered for 10 minutes in a cupful of boiling water. It is comforting for that tense, cramped sensation too: as is Lemon Balm, steeped in not quite- boiling water for 10 minutes. Prolonged or unexpected bleeding must be referred to a doctor.

Potter's P.M.T. Tablets are gently sedative, comforting to the uterine area, and soothing to that Pre-menstrual Tension: they contain Vervain, Gentian, Motherwort,

Meadow Anemone, Bearberry (to help counter toxic build-up) and Valerian.

Gerard House Helonias Compound Tablets were specially formulated to deal with the trials and tribulations of The Change - tension, hot flushes, fluid retention. Among other herbs they contain two which are well known tonics for the female reproductive system: Helonias Root, otherwise poetically known as False Unicorn Root, and Raspberry Leaves; together with Senna and Clivers to promote elimination problems, Parsley, Marshmallow, and tonic Centaury.

Migraine

Tension, food Allergies, the contraceptive Pill, anxiety, emotional stress and personality problems have all been studied as possible causes of the prostrating pattern headaches suffered by migraine victims, and it takes an expert practitioner to sort out individual cases and prescribe successfully. Stress seems particularly common: migraine sufferers are rarely affected on holiday. (See Nerves and Nervous Tension). Since poor diet is itself a major stress to the immune system, see also Allergies. Food allergies are now recognised even by orthodox medicine as a common cause. In a study at London's Hospital for Sick Children, 88 children with severe frequent migraine were put on diets to identify foods they were allergic to, and then on diets which eliminated them. 78 of them completely recovered on this diet, four improved greatly, and only six failed to respond. Commonest offending foods were cows' milk, egg, chocolate, orange and wheat: the artificial food colour tartrazine - E120 - was also often implicated. As well as advising on diet and general health, herbalists can call on a wide range of herbs to help remedy the underlying cause of the migraine and treat its more unpleasant symptoms. If your migraine attacks are severe, seek professional advice. If they're mild or infrequent, here are some remedies to try:

The big herbal success story in migraine is Feverfew, which appears to act by inhibiting or controlling the prostaglandin activity which gives rise to the pain and general malaise.

Controlled trials at a London hospital suggest that a 90-day course of four fresh leaves (make sure that it is the right species- *Tanacetum parthenium)* or about 200 mg daily could be effective in controlling the condition long-term. But this symptomatic treatment may leave the basic problem unresolved- and recurring; in which case it would be better to seek professional advice from a herbal practitioner. Some people have also suffered sore mouth or mouth ulcers while taking it. Potters Barefoot Brand Feverfew Tablets contain 200 mg of the herb, in a course of 90. Cinnamon and Ginger are both useful for countering the nausea common during a migraine attack: grate a little peeled fresh Ginger root, or add a pinch of dry Ginger to a cup of hot herbal tea.

Make up this mixture to deal with prostrating migraine headaches. It's made from two parts of Lemon Balm, to one part each of Wild Lettuce, Skullcap, Valerian Root - all soothing and sedative - and one part tonic, stimulating Rosemary. Try these; Lime Flower tea, Peppermint tea or Add a spike of dried Lavender to either of these to enhance their effect.

Certain essential oils of aromatic plants can be very helpful. Try rubbing into your forehead a few drops of any of the following: Lavender, Eucalyptus, Peppermint, Rosemary.

Since tension is almost always a feature of migraine, try any of the remedies listed under Nerves and Nervous Tension.

See also under Headaches.

Morning Sickness
The commonest cause of morning sickness (which can in fact strike at any time of the day during pregnancy) is junk food, according to an experienced practitioner friend of mine. If

you're eating a healthy diet with lots of wholegrain, vegetables, salads, fresh fruit; if you've cut out the tea, coffee, alcohol and cigarettes which mothers-to-be are now sternly warned against; and if you've cut right back on sugar, fried foods, white flour, you should sail happily through pregnancy with no problems. If you're eating healthily and you still get sick, check your vitamin intake - you may be low in Vitamin E or the B complex, in which case take brewer's yeast and wheat germ.

If that doesn't help, try a mild herbal remedy – hot Peppermint or Lime or Chamomile tea are all worth trying.

Meadowsweet might be better still. Steep a teaspoonful in a cupful of boiling water for ten minutes and take first thing in the morning - as you should, of course, all the others. Add a good pinch of dried Ginger or Cinnamon - both are highly effective against nausea; or pare off the thick skin of fresh ginger root, and grate a little of it into your herb tea.

And if that doesn't work and you're desperate, see a medical herbalist, who can check out the possible causes and prescribe mild but effective herbs that won't damage the unborn child.

See also Pregnancy

Mouth Ulcers

These painful little sores on the gums, inside the cheek or around the tongue may indicate a deficiency of vitamin C or the B Complex; they may be due to poor general health and lowered vitality; or they, can be a symptom of a food allergy. (See Allergies) If they persist, a general health overhaul by an expert practitioner is suggested.

For immediate relief, use a mouthwash of boiled water to which you have added some Tincture of Myrrh: 4-5 drops in a small glassful, holding it in the mouth as long as possible. Or tincture of Calendula: 4-5 drops in a small glassful. Or make an infusion of Sage: a teaspoonful of dried herb, rather more of the fresh leaves, infused covered in a cupful of boiling water for ten minutes.

Muscular Aches

Certain kinds of muscular ache - the dull ache in the small of the back known as lumbago, for instance - call for treatment by an osteopath, as do all forms of sciatica. Other aches and pains may be a form of rheumatism (see Rheumatism).

But odd aches and pains in the muscles, caused by sporting exertion, a pulled muscle, over-use of one set of muscles, too much bending and stooping as in gardening, can often be eased away by massage with the essential oil of one of a number of aromatic plants, or several in combination.

You can make up your own rubbing oil if you have fresh, or good dried plants. Rosemary, Lavender, and Thyme are among the most effective. Put the plant - a good fat sprig of it

- in a glass or enamel pan, pour over half a pint of olive or almond oil and heat gently until all the colour has left the plant. Throw it away, and your oil is ready, nice and warm.

You can also buy the essential oils from several suppliers - warm them before use. If olive or almond oil is beyond your purse, a good quality light vegetable oil will do.

There are many excellent ready-made remedies on the market. Tiger Balm, famous in the Far East for over half a century and brought back by many a traveller, is now available here in two formulations: White, containing Camphor,

Peppermint Oil, Cajuput Oil, Menthol and Clove Oil in a base of Paraffin; and Red, which is exactly the same except for the addition of Cassia Oil.

Potter's Nine Rubbing Oils is made from the following oils - Amber, Clove, Eucalyptus, Linseed, Wintergreen, Mustard, Turpentine, Thyme, Peppermint and Arachis.

Olbas Oil, containing Peppermint, Eucalyptus, Wintergreen, Cajuput, Clove and Juniper Berry Oils with Menthol, is another tried and trusted remedy.

Shirley Price's Massage Oil for aches and pains contains Juniper, Rosemary, Marjoram and Eucalyptus.

Weleda's Rheuma Ointment tackles the problem in another way - by powerfully stimulating local circulation to help counter inflammation and break up acid deposits: it contains Horse Chestnut Oil, Camphor, Larch Resin, Rosemary Oil and Basil, in an abrasive Sea-Salt based ointment. Gonne Pain Relieving Balm is another mix of aromatic oils:

Menthol, Camphor, Oil of Cajuput - specially valued in aromatherapy for local relief of rheumatic pain - Oil of Eucalyptus, Oil of Turpentine, and Methyl Salicylate. Its makers suggest that the part to be treated be first bathed in hot water, to open the pores and ensure deep penetration. In cases of fibrositis, vigorous massage should be avoided.

Cathay of Bournemouth make a Dragon Balm, a kingly mix of the healing aromatic oils: Camphor, Menthol, the Oils of Turpentine, Nutmeg, Eucalyptus, Cassia, Pine, together with

Thymol, Guaiacol and Balsam of Peru in a soft yellow paraffin base.

See also Feet, Rheumatism and Arthritis, Sprains Nerves and Nervous Tension Edginess, irritability and nervous tension are often treated by tranquillisers. Herbs offer a much more positive approach, that counters stress by toning the whole nervous system, while gently relaxing overstrung nerves. Since dependence on herbal tranquillisers, however, is just as unhealthy in the long run as dependence on a manmade one, herbs should be seen as a remedial measure, rather than a substitute for these powerful and perilous chemicals. The dangers of addiction to the benzodiazepine minor tranquillisers such as Ativan and Valium is now widely recognised, as is the cluster of painful mental and physical symptoms that can afflict those trying to withdraw from them. And it is here that herbs are more and more coming into their own, preferably prescribed for an individual case by a professional practitioner, using tried and tested nerve tonics or relaxants, such as Valerian, Motherwort, Scullcap.

For serious tensions or nervous problems, or to be weaned off dependence on benzodiazepine tranquillisers, consult a practitioner.

There are many useful herbal nerve tonics you can make for yourself, and several excellent ready-made ones, too. Any of the remedies listed under Depression will help counter stress and tension. Here are other useful ones:

Hops are so tranquillising that Gerard considered beer to be more of a medicine than an ordinary drink. Crush three of the little heads into a cup, cover with boiling water and steep, covered, for ten minutes. Hop pillows are a classic country remedy for nervous insomnia, and an agreeable way to give your nerves this particular tonic is to make a strong infusion of hops and pour it into a warm bedtime bath.

Valerian is the classic herbal nerve medicine, an ingredient in almost every prescription for nervous states. Its root – the valuable bit of it - smells odd and disagreeable, but the taste is not as bad, and if you add a little Peppermint, Lemon Balm or Vervain, together with a dash of honey, they will reinforce its action as well as improving its flavour. Take a teaspoon of the powdered root, with any other herb you wish, add a cupful of boiling water and steep, covered, for fifteen minutes. Valerian and other mild herbal sedatives are nutritive to nerves but like all drugs with a marked effect on the central nervous system they should not be taken for weeks on end. Since tea and coffee are high in caffeine, those suffering from nervous tension should avoid them as far as possible. Instead, drink Lime or Chamomile, both available in teabags, both delicious, both excellent for frayed nerves.

Bio-Strath Valerian Formula, in which Valerian is combined with Passionflower and Peppermint in the form of pleasanttasting drops. Excellent for pre-examination nerves.

Gerard House Natural Herb Nervine is good for stress and strain. Skullcap and Hops are combined with Asafoetida - which helps allay the digestive upsets that nervous problems can cause - together with Gentian and Valerian. Potter's Neurelax Tablets is another version of this classic five-herb formula.

Biophyllin tablets from Gerard House are excellent for nervous problems: combined in them are Valerian, Skullcap, soothing and sedative Passionflower, Jamaica Dogwood, and a touch of Cayenne to stimulate the circulation.

Potter's Ana-Sed helps soothe the aches and pains nervous tension can cause. It combines Hops, Jamaica Dogwood, Pasionflower, Pulsatilla and Wild Lettuce.

Salus Salusan Herbal Tonic is a sort of catch-all of over a dozen different herbs with a stimulating, strengthening influence on the nervous system and circulation. Among its ingredients are Passionflower, Lemon Balm, Hops, Hawthorn, St John's Wort and Barley Germ.

Weleda's Avena Sativa Compound is based on the sedative powers of Oats, with Hops, Passionflower and Valerian. Although it is calming and tranquillising, particularly helpful for those trying to wean themselves off dependency on Valium and synthetic 'downers', it doesn't knock you out during the daytime.

Lane's Quiet Life Tablets combine classic herbal calming agents - Valerian, Hops, Skullcap and Lettuce among them - with a dose of three B Vitamins - Bt, B2 and Nicotinic Acid.

Gerard House Valerian Compound contains herbs to strengthen the heart as well as ease tension. It combines Motherwort, Seaweed, Hops, Valerian, Wild Lettuce, Passionflower, Jamaica Dogwood and Skullcap.

Cathay of Bournemouth's Strong Thought, specifically for 'exam nerves', contains Hops and Valerian to calm those jitters, but also Dandelion to keep the system clean and toned- and Paprika, Ginger arid Pimento to boost mental alertness.

Like more and more herbal suppliers, Cathay also combine certain B Vitamins - Aneurin Hyd. Riboflavin and Nicotinamide- with tried and trusted herbal remedies for tension:

Motherwort, Hops, Vervain, Wild Lettuce, Passionflower, Lime tree and Skullcap, together with Kelp to supply minerals that may be deficient.

Napier's of Edinburgh combine Skullcap, Hops and Jamaica Dogwood with Indian Pennywort (valued by the American Indians) and Gentian for its tonic stimulant action, in their Assured Tablets. And yet another convenient nerve tonic tablet is Heath & Heather's Nerve Tablets - Skullcap, Hops and Valerian.

The aroma of certain plants can have a pronounced psychopharmacological effect, raising the spirits, calming anxiety and countering apathy and gloom. Among the essential oils which have this effect are those of Jasmine, Basil, Clary Sage, Lemon, Marjoram, Neroli. Add two or three drops to a warm - but not too hot - bedtime bath, in a warm bathroom; relax in it, breathing deeply, for ten minutes. Then blot yourself dry with a big towel and go straight to bed.

See also Depression, Insomnia, Post-natal Depression, Premenstrual Tension.

Nose Bleeds

Apply an ice-cold compress to the back of the neck - ice cubes wrapped in a tea towel, for instance and gently pinch the nostrils together.

After a minute or two, plug the nostrils gently with a plug of cotton wool soaked in either Lemon juice or distilled Witch-Hazel.

Frequent nosebleeds suggest that the tiny veins inside the nose are not very strong. Extra Vitamin C with bio-flavonoids and a course of Rutin Tablets will help.

In adults, nose bleeds may be a sign of high blood pressure and medical advice should be sought.

Piles

For badly swollen, bleeding or very painful piles (haemorrhoids) seek expert advice. For the milder sort which are chronic in an estimated fifty per cent of the population - swollen, occasionally unnoticed, sometimes a dull ache, very occasionally bleeding when a motion is passed - there is a specific herbal remedy, which the country-people who've used it down the centuries christened Pilewort, though you're more likely to know it as that cheerful little yellow spring flower, the Lesser Celandine. Both astringent and healing, Pilewort can do a marvellous job of shrinking and soothing those swollen and inflamed little veins in and around the anal passage.

They're due to congestion of the rectal veins, which can be caused by obstinate constipation, or by a sluggish liver. (A herbalist friend of mine has remarked that in many of her patients, it seems to be linked with eating a lot of cheese, particularly the blue-veined kind). See Constipation, Cut down on rich fatty foods, and step up your intake of fresh vegetables - particularly Celery, Artichoke, Spinach and Watercress, all terrific tonics for the liver. A course of Potter's

Lion Cleansing Herbs could be particularly useful, together with local applications of their Pilewort Green Ointment. Here are some other useful remedies.

Potter's Pilewort Compound for Haemorrhoids, which contains Pilewort, plus astringent and tonic Agrimony, and a dose of Senna and Cascara to help sort out your constipation problem.

Gerard House Pilewort Compound also has Pilewort, Senna and Cascara - but the extra astringency comes from Cranesbill Root.

Heath & Heather's Pile Tablets contain Stone Root, another traditional remedy for piles, together with healing and astringent Witch Hazel, Pilewort and some laxative Cascara. Potter's Pilewort Green Ointment. Calendula Ointment to soothe inflammation. Cold compresses of Witch Hazel, the colder the better - keep a bottle in the refrigerator.

Weleda's Hammamelis Folium (Witch Hazel Leaf) Ointment, and suppositories could be used. If poor general circulation could be one explanation for your piles, take a regular supplement of Rutin Tablets to strengthen veins and capillaries.

Post-Natal Depression

It would be astonishing if most women *didn't* suffer from some degree of low spirits in the days and sometimes weeks after their baby is born. They've often been made a lovely fuss of while they were pregnant, they've been waited on hand and foot for a blissful few days in hospital while somebody else did all the worrying - and suddenly they're home, the baby is the centre of attention, the sense of anticlimax is crushing, there's a pile of dirty nappies that never gets smaller, their husband wants his supper on the table just as usual, they're worried sick about the new baby half the time, they don't have time to eat properly so they snatch at a sandwich or a biscuit - and they're averaging maybe five hours of broken sleep a night. So who wouldn't get depressed? Add to all that the vast hormonal adjustments their weary body is trying to make, and that's post-natal depression. For really severe Depression medical help must be sought immediately.

Much postnatal depression may result from low levels of zinc. Pregnant women and nursing mothers have particularly high needs for this mineral- around 25 mg daily compared to 12-15 mg for ordinary adults - an amount seldom supplied by an ordinary diet. Take a supplement supplying at least this amount of zinc, together with plenty of vitamins C and B6.

Diet is ultra-important: the woman suffering from this rundown, weepy state needs plenty of good nourishing food, fresh fruit and vegetables, milk, cheese, yogurt to rebuild her strength. She's likely to be low in B vitamins - of which brewers' yeast is much the best source. (I found that a palatable way to take it was to put a dessertspoonful in the blender with a couple of big spoons of yogurt, a cupful of milk, and a sliced banana, for a big milk shake with a nutty but perfectly pleasant flavour.)

She's certainly in need of a good tonic (See Convalescence).

The following herbs and spices have the advantage not only of being readily available in the well-stocked spice rack, but of helping to stimulate the milk flow if she is breastfeeding:

Fennel, Cumin, Caraway or Dill seeds. Take a teaspoon of any one of them, crush them (with a rolling-pin between two layers of greaseproof paper or foil is as good a way as any), pour a cupful of boiling water over them and steep, covered, for ten minutes. This ·warm spicy tea should be drunk two or three times a day, perhaps sweetened with a little honey. Fenugreek tea may be made the same way, and is equally stimulating to the milk supply and tonic to the spirits. Don't try crushing the seeds, simply infuse them for fifteen minutes.

Raspberry Leaf Tea not -only helps ease childbirth, it's a marvellous tonic - to the system generally and to the whole uterine area in particular. A teaspoon to a cupful of boiling water, infused covered 10 minutes, and drunk warm three times a day, will help tone and strengthen the tired muscles of womb and vagina. For other suggestions, see Depression.

Many of the herb remedies most effective for countering it are also nutritious, such as Oats.

Pregnancy

Herbal medicine, other than the mildest of herbal teas, is best avoided during pregnancy, like all other medicines. The great exception is Raspberry Leaf, which has a long tradition of folk use - and an 'equally impressive modern reputation among herbalists - as a marvellous aid to easy childbirth, toning and bracing the whole reproductive system and its muscles. It should be taken for three months beforehand: 1ounce (30 g) of the dried herb to a 1pint (550 ml) of water, infused covered for fifteen minutes, sweetened if you like with a little honey and drunk warm two or three times a day, a cupful at a time.

Tablets of Raspberry Leaf are supplied by Baldwin's, and many women will find them more convenient to take - certainly in hospital, where they should be continued right up to the onset of labour. Afterwards, they make an excellent post-natal tonic, to help restore normal function and tone.

Note Athletic women, with muscles in splendid shape, should consult a herbal practitioner before taking Raspberry Leaf, because it is possible to over-tone the muscles of the reproductive system and a prolonged labour could result.

See also Breastfeeding Problems, Post-natal Depression.

Rheumatism and Arthritis

Every year millions of people consult their doctors about rheumatic ailments, the assorted aches and pains arising out of inflamed joints or muscle tissue, and wear-and-tear around the joints, which can vary from an occasional twinge to the deep seated, agonising and sometimes crippling pain for which even the most powerful painkillers of orthodox medicine can bring little more than transient relief.

A skilled herbal practitioner will make a detailed study of a patient's medical history to work out the form his particular rheumatic ailment takes, what caused it, and how to control or overcome it before he prescribes from a wide range of useful herbs to treat the underlying condition and restore the patient to health and activity.

In all forms of rheumatic disease, there are two main causes: stress, tension and personality problems of one form or another, which can disturb the delicate hormonal and chemical balance of the system, and a poor, inadequate diet, laced with chemical additives and deficient in vitamins and minerals. Some forms of arthritis are triggered by injury to joints or spine, and may need treatment from a qualified osteopath to correct the underlying lesion. Food or chemical sensitivities are more and more being seen as culprits in many cases of arthritis: on diets eliminating foods to which they were susceptible - wheat and milk as usual are common offenders - arthritic patients have often made complete recoveries from agonising stiffness and joint pain. See Allergies.

Constipation is almost always a factor in rheumatic disease, causing toxic overload which may pile up as acid deposits in joints or muscles, so most herbal prescriptions for these conditions include either herbs which promote mild perspiration - Guaiacum or Prickly Ash, or which help to cleanse the blood and are laxative or diuretic, such as Dandelion, Rhubarb or Bearberry (see also Constipation.)

Herbalists can prescribe many other useful herbs. Some deal with stress (see Nerves) and nourish the nerves, others counter swelling and irritation, and there are herbs that stimulate the circulation to promote healing of bone and tissue. They will also prescribe herbs to allay and soothe arthritic pain. In the therapeutic doses used by herbalists, these are almost invariably free of the side-effects so common with orthodox painkilling drugs. Herbalists will also advise on an acid-free diet crucial to the treatment of these disorders.

Common to almost all the diets found helpful in arthritis and rheumatism are the following suggestions. No tea, coffee, alcohol or white sugar. You can eat fish and chicken, but not red meat, Acid fruits such as oranges, strawberries and rhubarb are out, but lemons are allowed and, indeed, highly recommended. Use wholegrain rather than white flour and, if possible, avoid any processed foods containing synthetic additives. For some people no dairy foods - butter, cheese, milk, yogurt - are permitted, although calcium and Vitamins A and D supplements will be necessary to replace those normally supplied by dairy foods. Vitamin and mineral intake should be more than adequate; zinc may be particularly important - it may be worth taking the zinc test described under Anorexia. So are the B vitamins. And plenty of exercise or at least gentle walking is always advised to stimulate the circulation and aid relaxation. Without a basic fitness programme of this kind, the most wonderful herbal remedies in the world won't be much good.

The great twentieth-century discovery for the treatment of arthritis and rheumatism has been a plant found in central southern Africa, *Harpagophytum procumbens,* called Devil's Claw after the vicious down-curving thorns that can cripple the unwary human or animal that treads on it. This fact perhaps suggested to the local tribesmen that it might be effective against the crippling pains of rheumatism and arthritis, and in dozens of trials conducted - mainly in Germany, it has been shown to be precisely that. It is the dried and powdered tubers that are used. Their action seems to be both detoxifying and stimulating to the body's own immune system; and no harmful effects have so far shown up even in high doses, and after months of use. Like all herbal treatment for chronic illnesses it should be persisted with for two or three weeks before effects can be expected to show up, and thereafter continued for eight to nine weeks at a time, although - again as with remedies for chronic disorders - it's a good idea to give your body a break from the treatment after each course.

I suggest intervals of three weeks at a time. However, Diabetics should not take Devil's Claw except under medical supervision, since it can significantly lower the dose of insulin they need, and they might find themselves overdosing with insulin, which could be dangerous. Herbal practitioners have found that although Devil's Claw works marvellously for some people, it's much less effective for others. So if you feel no benefit at all after a month, discontinue it, and switch to something else. Devil's Claw is available in tablet or teabag form.

Celery Seeds, whose high alkaline value helps to counter acid formation in the blood and clear it out of the system. You can buy Celery-Seed Capsules or tablets (from Heath & Heather) and drink Biotta Celery Juice. Celery Seeds are a component of some of the most effective herbal remedies for rheumatism on the market - or you can simply eat plenty of Celery. In Romany medicine, Celery is stewed in milk for half an hour or so, then the milk is drunk and the Celery eaten.

Nettles are also highly effective for rheumatism. Appropriately it's the Stinging Nettle that is so good at countering the stinging pains of rheumatic disorders. Nettles, like Celery, are highly alkaline, and attack excess acid in the system. They are rich in iron, excellent for the circulation, and they contain tonic quantities of other useful minerals and vitamins. The valuable part is the top of the young nettle, which can be gathered in spring or summer from any handy patch of wasteland. Make sure, though, that it's not getting a dose of pesticide from a neighbouring crop, or lead contamination from the exhausts of passing cars. Wash it carefully before use.

The young Nettle tops can be used as one ingredient in a green soup, or stewed like' spinach, which they slightly resemble - but drink the water, too. You can buy Nettle teabags from a health-food shop if you're city-bound, or make your own infusion from dried Nettle Tops bought from a herbal supplier. Both Celery and Nettles are combined, together with Birch - an effective diuretic - in Hofels' Herb Formula R tablets.

Poor circulation is a factor in some kinds of rheumatism. An excellent remedy for this is the bark or berries of the Prickly Ash tree, highly prized by the American Indians as a remedy for rheumatism and a marvellous cleanser of the blood, and later adopted by white settlers. You can buy Prickly Ash tablets from Gerard House. Prickly Ash *ifs* also an ingredient of one of the most enduringly popular and successful herbal remedies ever - formulared in this country: Potter's Tabritis - until recently known as Arthritabs. In table~ is a combination of herbs which helps to cleanse and detoxify the entire system and relieve the pain of inflamed joints and muscles. It comprises Elder Flowers and Yarrow for their anti-inflammatory action, Poke Root, Poplar Bark and Prickly Ash for their antirheumatic properties, and Senna Leaves, Bearberry, Clivers and Burdock to promote elimination.

Guaiacum, or the heartwood of the *Lignum vitae* tree found in the West Indies, was for long considered a cure for syphilis.

Today, it's one of the first herbs that professional practitioners turn to in the treatment of chronic rheumatism or rheumatoid arthritis. It is combined with other anti-rheumatic tonic and cleansing herbs - White Willow, White Poplar Bark, Black Cohosh, Sarsaparilla and Rhubarb - in Ligvite Tablets, from Gerard House. '

White Willow contains salicin, which the body converts into salicylic acid. A synthetic derivative of this, acetylsalicylic acid, is today's most commonly swallowed drug - aspirin – and doctors often turn to it first for the relief of rheumatic pain and inflammation. White Willow has the same anti-inflammatory and painkilling properties, without the toxic side effects which can result from even quite small doses of aspirin, and it is another obvious choice for professional herbalists treating rheumatoid arthritis, particularly when there is much pain and inflammation. It is often combined with Black Cohosh, Celery and Guaiacum. So take Ligvites from Gerard House - and eat plenty of Celery.

Another excellent formula comes from the Edinburgh herbalists, Napier's. Their Rheumatic Tablets contain the great antirheumatics Poke Root and Black Cohosh, plus Guaiacum Resin, Burdock, Sarsaparilla, Prickly Ash and Cayenne.

In the course of clinical trials designed to test the various Bio-Strath formulae, it was found - to everybody's surprise that the common Cowslip, *Primula veris,* was even more effective in allaying rheumatic pain and inflammation than White Willow. Both Cowslip and White Willow, accordingly, were combined with the tonic herbal base of Bio-Strath in their Willow Formula.

Another formula containing Guaiacum is Heath' & Heather's Rheumatic Pain Tablets, which also have a dash of Capsicum Oleoresin to stimulate the circulation, and Rhubarb, Bearberry, Bogbean and Celery Seed for detoxification and elimination of waste matter.

Seaweed is a rich source of many important trace elements, often lacking even in a well-balanced diet, and particularly important to those who suffer from degenerative diseases such as Arthritis. There are many excellent Kelp or Seaweed tablets on the market. One of the best is Fjord brand, which contains two varieties of Seaweed from a remote Norwegian fjord. They can be ordered by post, in containers of 200 capsules. Potters new Tabritis Plus tablets have kelp added to their excellent Tabritis Formula. Lemons taste so particularly acid that it's natural to assume there can be no place for them in a diet designed to combat excess acidity, such as is strongly recommended to all arthritic sufferers. In fact as recent research in France has shown, the natural citric acid they contain is oxidised during digestion, and the remaining salts yield carbonates and bicarbonates of both calcium and potassium, which maintain the alkalinity of the blood and counter excess acidity. So the juice of a whole Lemon squeezed into a glass of warm water first thing every morning is not only a tonic to your liver, but will help to counter acidity too.

Onions, with their high vitamin and mineral content and their diuretic properties, are a particularly useful foodstuff for rheumatic sufferers. Eat them in your daily diet, or as a drink in the form of a decoction. Add three chopped, unpeeled (but carefully washed) Onions to 1Y4 pints (1 litre) of water. Boil for fifteen minutes, then strain. Drink a glass first thing in the morning and last thing at night.

Soothing baths

Most rheumatic sufferers know the relief that Epsom salts added to a hot bath can bring to their pain and stiffness. A strong infusion of aromatic plants can be equally tonic, helping to soothe away aches and pains. Weleda make Rosemary, Pine or Lavender Bath, each containing the pure essential plant oils. All three are used for rheumatic ailments in

French aromatherapy, to stimulate the circulation locally and generally, and bring comforting warmth to aching limbs. Use a Rosemary bath in the morning, since it is invigorating, a Pine or Lavender bath at night-time for relaxation. To make your own aromatic bath, take a big bunch of fresh or dried Thyme, add it to a pan containing two pints (1 litre) of boiling water, simmer for twenty minutes, covered, strain, and add to a hot bath.

Seaweed baths are a marvellous way to absorb a dose of all the minerals and trace-elements found in seaweed, in which rheumatic sufferers are often deficient. They are also very soothing for arthritic pain, Ground Seaweed Bath is one way to give yourself this treatment, which now features in expensive spas.

Aromatic Rubs

Painfully inflamed, hot and aching joints can be eased by rubbing in aromatic plant oils. Chamomile is one of the most effective: add an ounce (30 g) of the dried flower heads to 10 tablespoons of pure olive (or other vegetable) oil, and heat, covered, over a saucepan of simmering water for two hours.

Strain through fine muslin or cheesecloth. Thyme, Rosemary or Bay Leaves can be used in the same way to make a fragrant and soothing rubbing oil. Aroma therapists make a soothing rub which contains Juniper, Rosemary and Marjoram.

For other-suggestions, see Muscular Aches and Pains:

Any of the rubbing oils suggested there will help.

Shingles

The maddening itching, or the deep aching pain of shingles is the work of the *herpes zoster* virus, which can live on harmlessly in your body for years following an early attack of chicken pox. A tired, run-down condition, acute nervous or emotional tension, even excessive heat, can bring the dormant virus to life, and inflamed major sensory nerves are the result. These are characteristically on and around the chest or trunk, but also occur on the head, hands, thighs or occasionally knees. The underlying condition needs careful diagnosis, and should be treated by a professional herbal practitioner, who can prescribe herbs to improve your general resistance, nourish and tone the nervous system, and allay the inflammation that makes life temporarily so unbearable. Here are some remedies.

If you're run down, poorly, tired, see Convalescence for a good tonic. To help you combat nervous or emotional strain, see Nerves. To allay pain and itching, try one of the following:

The herbal practitioner may well suggest that you apply

Vitamin E oil to the lesions - you can prick capsules of the pure oil and squeeze it out.

A cold compress made with a teaspoon of Tincture of Hypericum in a cupful of water. Hypericum is particularly" soothing to injured nerves and the resulting pain. A cold compress made in the same way with Tincture of Calendula, 'or the two combined in Hypercal, from Nelson's.

Calendula, Hypericum or Chickweed Ointment may also be effective.

Make an infusion of Chamomile, strain and cool it, and apply it as a compress.

Weleda's Combudoron Lotion is made from extracts of *Urtica urens,* the Lesser Nettle, with a little Arnica. Dilute a teaspoon in a cupful of cold water, and apply as a cold compress.

Thornham Herbs make a Four Thieves' Vinegar, after a classic French formula. The essential oils of Sage, Thyme, Rosemary and Lavender are added to distilled water. Swab the affected areas gently with this.

Oil of Evening Primrose has also been found effective (see "Eczema).

Shock

The best remedy I know for shock is Dr Bach's Rescue Remedy. It comes in a small dropper bottle which I carry with me everywhere - as does anyone who has learned what a marvellous remedy it is. It's on-the-spot, safe, easy-to administer first aid for any degree of shock, from the mild case following a child's nasty tumble to the severe shock – which can be life-threatening - following serious injury, burns, electrocution, etc. If the patient is conscious, put four or five drops on his tongue. If unconscious, moisten his lips with it.

Dr Edward Bach (1880-1936) was a successful London bacteriologist till he threw up a good job to go herb-hunting.

He was convinced that most diseases were the result of mental or emotional disturbances or weakness, and he looked for plants that could cure these, soaking the ones he chose in pure spring water that was left to stand in the full spring sunshine.

Remedies for five of these states of negative emotion - including terror, shock and fear of death, were combined in what he called his Rescue Remedy. And if all this sounds to you like the worst excesses of medieval mumbo-jumbo, all I can say is - try it next time someone in your family has a bad accident, or receives extremely bad news - or a child has to submit to a painful operation. It contains a small quantity of alcohol, so should not be given to anyone you suspect of being a cured alcoholic. The ingredients are: Star of Bethlehem for shock; Rock Rose for terror and panic, Impatiens for mental stress, Cherry Plum for despair and Clematis for faintness and confusion. "Potter's Antispasmodic Drops are based on a formula that goes back at least to the nineteenth century. Made from herbs" with potent antispasmodic and sedative action – including Valerian

Root, Scullcap, Lobelia, Black Cohosh Root, Fennel and Cayenne - it was successfully used by Victorian practitioners, even in cases of lockjaw and convulsions.

Skin Problems

Skin problems such as acne, eczema, dermatitis or psoriasis may have a variety of causes, ranging through hormonal imbalance "or stress to external allergens or adverse drug reactions. But nutritional deficiencies and a poor diet high in junk foods will certainly aggravate them. And although conventional suppressive treatment - cortisone creams, peeling or abrasion, ultra-violet ray or X-ray therapy, or courses of hormones or antibiotics - may bring a welcome respite, they can have most unwelcome side effects, while the problems themselves may recur after a time. The object of the herbalist is to restore the body to its normal healthy function, so that its own immune system can cope efficiently with the problem. Thus he will give careful advice on diet and life style, as well as prescribing blood-cleansing and tonic herbs that will relieve constipation, counter inflammation and infection, calm stress, and tone up all the systems of the body. If your skin problems don't yield to the home treatments suggested here," take them to a trained herbal practitioner for expert attention.

Check your vitamin and mineral intake and, if necessary, take supplements. Vitamins A, B complex, C and E are all stressed. A good Seaweed pill is a natural source of most important minerals, but Zinc in particular is seen more and more as a key nutrient in skin health, and it is poorly supplied in the products of modern agriculture with its artificial fertilisers and pesticides.

Skin problems call for kitchen medicine in the form of a correct diet. Cut out sugar and refined carbohydrates, substitute vegetable oils for dairy fats as far as possible, eat chicken or fish in preference to meat, cut down on alcohol, soft drinks, tea and coffee, and drink mineral water or herbal tisanes instead - Chamomile, Lime and Peppermint. Eat plenty of fruit, nuts, sprouted seeds, salads and green vegetables. The following are particularly useful since they're important natural sources of blood-cleansing minerals such as iron, sulphur, potassium: Radishes with their green tops, Parsley, Celery, young Dandelion Leaves, Spinach, Carrots, Watercress, Green Pepper, Spring Onions. They're particularly good in small doses of concentrated juice from the raw vegetable, and blending them is much easier than fiddling about with a juicer (which most people don't possess anyway).

Make an assortment of three or four vegetables, and chop them roughly - there should be enough to fill about half a cup.

Drop them in the blender with a cupful of water, preferably uncarbonated mineral water, and blend for a couple of minutes. The result is thick raw vegetable soup, absolutely delicious and fresh to taste, which can be varied from day to day so that it never tastes the same. Have a glassful- no moreonce a day, and eat as much as you like of the same vegetables in salad form.

The Biotta range of vegetable juices includes Celery, Beetroot and Carrot, all made from organically-grown vegetables.

Constipation is almost always a factor in skin problems. The following herbs are known as alteratives, useful for treating all toxicities of the blood, infections, skin eruptions, and favourably 'altering' the entire system. The classic alteratives used in skin problems are Dandelion, Burdock, Yellow Dock, Echinacea, Chaparral, Sarsaparilla, Nettles and Red Clover. There are" so many excellent blood-purifying formulas made up into tablet or elixir form and readily available in health-food stores or by direct mail order, that it's hardly worth bothering to track down the different herbs for making up your own special blood-purifying mixture. The made-up formulas are likely to be cheaper into the bargain.

Among the best of them are: Muir's Blu Glan Tablets contain traditional alteratives - Yellow Dock, Burdock, Echinacea, Red Clover and Sarsa parilla plus tonic Vervain and a little laxative Senna.

Blue Flag Root Tablets, from Gerard House, are designed to fortify the blood and help to adjust glandular imbalance. As well as Blue Flag Root, they contain Queen's Delight, Poke Root, Sarsaparilla, and Burdock Root.

Blue Flag - both laxative and diuretic, with a marked action in skin problems - is an ingredient in Heath & Heather's Blood Purifying Mixture, to be taken by the teaspoonful in water. Its other ingredients are Burdock, Red Clover, Yellow Dock, Echinacea, a spot of laxative Senna, and a dash of Cayenne.

Their Blood Purifying Tablets have a strong diuretic action: they contain Fumitory, Burdock, Buckbean, Clivers and Senna Leaf.

One of the best alternatives in any skin problem is Echinacea, whose antibiotic properties are being studied with increasing interest, as are its powers to stimulate the body's own healing mechanisms. You can buy it in the form of a tincture made from the whole fresh plant, called Echinaforce, by Dr Vogel's Bioforce Company. Or you can take a course of Echinacea Tablets: Baldwin's, Potter's, Gerard House supply these.

(Potter's tablets are called Skin Clear).

Echinacea is combined with another natural antibiotic, Chaparral, together with Ginseng, to counter stress and tension, available in tablet form from Gerard House.

Stress is almost a factor in skin problems - often one cause of them and almost invariably a consequence, particularly in luckless teenagers suffering disfiguring Acne. See under Nerves and Nervous Tension.

Vital to those suffering from skin problems are regular vigorous exercise, to stimulate the circulation, and plenty of fresh air, since the ultra-violet light that is present even on grey cloudy days is beneficial to the skin - too much strong sunshine, on the other hand, is not.

Sinusitis

Inflammation of the mucous membrane lining the sinus cavities that open into the nose can be acutely painful, often causing a constant dull headache that occasionally becomes acute, and a painful stuffed-up feeling. Check for an allergy problem, particularly with cows' milk and dairy products: see section on Allergies. Sinus problems often follow a cold when the mucous membrane in the sinus passages becomes irritated and inflamed, and infection sets in. See Catarrh. Any of these remedies will help to clear the blocked passages. Inhalations of Menthol, Olbas Oil, or Tincture of Benzoin (ask for Friar's Balsam at the chemist) will all help. Try gentle steaming: make a strong infusion of Chamomile Flowers and add it to the water; or add a few drops of the essential oil of Lavender, Eucalyptus, Pine or Thyme.

A few drops of Lemon juice put into the nostrils out of a dropper, and sniffed back up into the head - very gently – will counter infection. For the first few minutes you may feel that the cure is worse than the complaint, but the marvellous clearheaded feeling that follows is well worth it. And a course of Potter's Antifect should clear it completely. It could take three to four weeks.

Spanish Tummy

Too much alcohol, too much sun, too much ripe fruit, doubtful drinking water, dubious shellfish or meat, fish past its fresh prime, involuntary swallows of the heavily polluted Mediterranean while bathing, funny chemicals in the cheap local vino, and heavy pesticide contamination of. unwashed fruit or vegetables (the Spanish are particularly trigger-happy with these) - anyone of these holiday hazards can bring on the nausea, the griping stomach pains, the prostration, and often the vile, racking headache of the authentic Spanish Tummy.

Some people settle it with a good stiff brandy, others swear by Dr Collis-Browne's Chlorodyne, others by kaolin and morphine mixtures. For mild cases, try any of the remedies listed under Diarrhoea.

For the real horror, forewarned is forearmed - travel with one of the following, plus a supply of vegetable Charcoal tablets. This useful substance absorbs toxic gases and waste on 'its way down the alimentary canal, carrying them safely out of the body. Take a couple every two hours or so.

Potter's Spanish Tummy Mixture will help calm and soothe the intestinal tract. Made from powerfully astringent herbs - Blackberry Root Bark and Gum Catechu, it should soothe the griping pangs.

Papaya Tablets from Gerard House are a useful mix: Papaya for its ability to break down undigested proteins in the digestive and intestinal tract, Charcoal, Slippery Elm to soothe and heal irritated mucous membrane, and Goldenseal for its cleansing, tonic powers.

Potter's Acidosis Tablets, containing Meadowsweet, to purify and tone the intestinal tract, are also useful.

Travellers who beg the waiter to serve them their food without 'all that awful garlic' are rejecting very effective preventative medicine in this case, since Garlic is a potent bactericide. Swallowing a 'One a Day' Garlic Pill every morning could be the best way to ensure a tummy trouble- free holiday. A few drops of Lemon juice in doubtful 'water (if you can't get bottled spring water) or added to fish or meat are added protection - like Garlic, Lemon is a useful bactericide. Avoid dehydration by drinking plenty of boiled or mineral water, with a little lemon juice added if possible.

Travellers in more exotic places such as the Far East and Central and South America should be aware that what may seem like a violent attack of food poisoning may in fact be the start of something much more serious, such as dysentery, hepatitis or one of the Typhoid group. Any of these remedies will help alleviate the symptoms, but reliable medical help should be procured as soon as possible.

Splinters'
A good 'drawing' ointment is what you need to loosen these painful fragments of wood or thorn underneath the skin or nails. Marshmallow or Comfrey, or the two combined in one ointment: Potter's make a Brown Marshmallow Ointment, or a Mallow and Slippery Elm Drawing Ointment. Gerard House have a Marshmallow and Slippery Elm Ointment. Soak the affected part in hot water, pat dry, smear the ointment thickly over it,

and put a dressing on top to keep it in place. Sea-urchin spines can be treated the same way.

A hot poultice of powdered Slippery Elm or powdered Comfrey Root, moistened with hot water, or an infusion of the respective herbs, is equally good, if more fuss.

Sprains and Fractures

If there is the slightest chance that the affected limb is fractured seek professional advice, including an X-ray, immediately. Meanwhile, hot compresses applied *gently* to the affected area will help to reduce both pain and swelling by stimulating local circulation. Hot water will do splendidly but strong Comfrey tea would be better still.

Comfrey Oil or Ointment gently stroked into the area will also give relief.

Arnica is well known for its usefulness in sprains or bruises use an ointment, or add a few drops of Tincture of Arnica to a cupful of warm water. (Don't use Tincture of Arnica neat on the skin as it can set up local irritation, and don't use it on injuries where the skin is broken.)

Witch Hazel helps to counter swelling and inflammation - use it for compresses, or soak the bandage in it.

See also Shock.

Sore Throat

A gargle of Red Sage tea is so wonderful a remedy for a sore throat, and so rapid in the relief it brings, that I am never without a packet of dried Sage leaves in my first-aid cupboard.

Infuse a teaspoonful in a cup of boiling water, covered, for ten minutes. Add a dash of vinegar. Gargle, holding your head right back and keeping it in contact with the inflamed throat for as long as possible. You can drink the rest - not more than a couple of cups a day, taken half a cup at a time. It is excellent for both colds and 'flu - often associated with sore throats.

If you have no Sage, gargle with hot water into which you have squeezed the juice of a Lemon. Add honey if you like – and drink the rest.

Thyme tea is also good for a sore throat. Infuse a teaspoon of dried, or rather more of fresh, Thyme, in a cupful of boiling water for ten minutes, covered. Gargle with it as hot as you can; drink half a cupful, warm, three times a day for general cold and 'flu relief. Hot Sage or Thyme tea, made by infusing a teaspoon of the dried herb, or more of the fresh, in a cupful of boiling water, covered, for ten minutes, can be used as a compress. Dip a clean cotton scarf in the hot tea, wring it out, and wrap it around the throat. Cover it with another scarf to keep it in place.

See also Colds, Influenza, Laryngitis, Tonsillitis.

Styes. See under Conjunctivitis.

Sunburn

Any of the remedies suggested under Burns will be helpful, and the same principle applies: cool the sunburned area as quickly as possible, before applying anything.A useful remedy available on most Mediterranean beaches is Chamomile tea - Manzanilla in Spain. Allow it to cool, and wash burned parts with it. For extra-fast relief, pierce and squeeze Vitamin E capsules onto the burned area, or add the oil to any soothing ointment you may apply.

Too much sun is dehydrating and victims of bad sunburn should drink plenty of water. If they seem seriously affected, treat for shock - see under Shock and send for medical help.

Tonsillitis

For acute tonsillitis, with Fever, seek professional advice, especially in the case of children.

For milder cases, or while you're waiting for expert help to arrive, put the patient to bed and treat for Fever. Make a gargle of hot Sage or Thyme tea, (see Sore Throat), and make them gargle at least once an hour. If you have neither Sage nor Thyme, use pure Lemon Juice, freshly squeezed and used neat, or diluted with a little warm water. Cold compresses of Thyme or Sage tea should be applied to the throat, lightly bandaged into place and wrapped around with a silk scarf. Or gently rub a little Garlic Oil into the throat, wrapping lint or a scarf round it.

To help combat general infection, take a course of Echinacea Tablets, Echinaforce Drops, or Potter's Antifect, in which Echinacea is combined with Garlic, together with a little medicinal Charcoal to counter possible digestive problems in those who are sensitive to Garlic.

See also Fever, Sore Throat.

Toothache

Prevention is the best cure, but nobody would be so cruel as to point this out to a victim of the agonies of toothache, which tends to strike late in the evening or at the weekend, when dentists are not on call unless you live near a dental hospital.

Try any of the following remedies, but if you don't have them in the house, any chemist (and there's usually one open at night and weekends in major centres) should stock Oil of Cloves.

The pain comes from the throbbing inflammation following infection of the tooth or gums. To counter it, chew on a clove of Garlic - powerfully anti-infective - or on a Clove, which is not just anti-infective, but has a remarkable local anaesthetic action into the bargain. (In Germany, they've now developed a general anaesthetic based on Cloves). If you have oil of Cloves, soak a cotton wool bud in it, or a little cotton wool wound round the tip of an orange stick, and massage the gum around the aching tooth.

Tincture of Calendula is marvellous first aid: soak a plug of cotton wool in a strong lotion - half a teaspoon to an egg cupful of boiled water - and pack it around the infected gum or into the cavity.

Make an infusion of Thyme or Sage: a teaspoonful steeped, covered, for ten minutes in a cupful of boiling water. Swill it repeatedly around the mouth. Both Thyme and Sage will help to counter infection and inflammation, and the heat is soothing to pain.

If you have either in the house, Potter's Ana-Sed or Herbprin - both formulated from plants that have sedative, anodyne or painkilling properties - would help. So would a dozen drops of Potter's Antispasmodic Drops in a small glass of water.

See also Gums.

Travel Sickness

A combination of travel nerves and upset stomach produces the dreadful nausea or discomfort which can make a sea voyage a nightmare for many people. A herbal remedy, powdered Ginger Root, had proved superior in the treatment of this condition.

This is not always easy to take so you can order Tincture of Ginger from Baldwin's, and take a small bottle of it with you, to be administered 10 drops at a time in a little water for adults, and 2-3 drops well diluted in warm water for children.

Many greengrocers and supermarkets sell fresh Ginger root nowadays. Peel it, and grate a little into hot Chamomile tea.

Take this in a small thermos flask for the journey: sweeten with a little honey.

Or you can buy Healthcrafts' Travel Well Tablets, which contain extract of African Ginger, together with two herbs with a comforting action on the stomach+ Chamomile and Meadowsweet, plus a little Vitamin B6 to calm travel nerves.

If you feel that fear is the true course of your travel sickness see under Nerves for some effective remedies.

Cat hay .of Bournemouth also tackle the problem on both fronts - physiological and psychological: their Travel Sickness Tablets contain Valerian, Hops and Skullcap for their sedative action, Gum, Asafetida to calm that heaving stomach, and Gentian to give it tonic comfort.

Ulcers, Gastric and Duodenal

Ulcers in the lining of the stomach (gastric) or the duodenum (duodenal) develop when excess acid secreted by the stomach eats its way into the mucous membrane lining. The earliest symptoms are stomach-ache, nausea, heartburn; as the ulcer develops, it is characterised by intense gnawing pain. Apart from the agony, ulcers can inflict fearsome damage: anaemia from haemorrhaging and subsequent loss of blood, damage and scarring to the stomach and duodenum lining. And acid leaking through the ulcer can eat its way into the peritoneum, the membrane lining in the stomach cavity - which will almost inevitably cause severe bacterial infection and be life threatening.

The classic triggers of gastric and duodenal ulcers are stress and tension, combined with a diet high in rich fatty foods, refined carbohydrates and alcohol - typically the successful executive's disease. Smoking may cause some ulcers, and certainly makes them worse - some can be cured just by stopping smoking. Coffee and tea - gastro-intestinal irritants - can exacerbate them too. So can aspirin, which should never be taken by ulcer sufferers. Check the possibility that a food Allergy is responsible: the milk heavily featured in the bland diets prescribed for ulcers has often proved to be the actual cause when carefully investigated.

Ulcers are so painful, and their potential for damage is so severe, that medical advice should be sought as soon as they are suspected. Conventional treatment relies heavily on drugs that will check excess production of gastric acid and antacids to reduce or neutralise it - which certainly bring wonderful relief, but leave the basic problem unresolved. The herbal practitioner will suggest a special diet that may be severely restrictive at first, to help eliminate the condition that allowed the ulcer to develop in the first place; and he will prescribe herbs that will help combat tension, normalise the function of the entire digestive system, and soothe and heal the inflamed mucous membrane lining stomach and duodenum.

See under Nerves and Nervous Tension for suggestions on coping with stress. To help restore normal healthy function to your stomach, see under Digestive Disorders.

Here are some simple remedies:

An infusion of Lemon Balm - a teaspoon infused 15 minutes, covered, in a cupful of not quite boiling water - is, as its name suggests, comforting to the poor suffering stomach.

An infusion of Chamomile is soothing, comforting and healing: a teaspoon of the dried florets infused covered in a cupful of boiling water for 10 minutes.

Tonic Fenugreek will help repair damage and promote healthy function in your digestive system; crush an ounce of the seeds (with a rolling pin, between layers of greaseproof paper) and simmer them covered for la minutes in a pint of water. Drink a cupful three times a day, before meals.

The two herbal remedies for gastric and duodenal ulcers – as you might expect - are Slippery Elm Bark and Marshmallow Root; with their high mucilage content, they are soothing and healing to the entire digestive tract, and a marvellous remedy, therefore, for the dreadful pain. Both Slippery Elm and Marshmallow Root can be taken three times a day, between meals or whenever the pain is particularly severe. As well as medicine, Slippery Elm is also food: complete nourishment for an invalid.

Raw vegetable juices· are particularly helpful in the treatment of ulcers: Celery or Carrot juice, made from organically grown vegetables.

See also Digestive Problems, Mouth Ulcers.

Ulcers: External

Persistent ulcers that refuse to heal need expert attention: chronic varicose ulcers can be particularly resistant to treatment. A qualified herbal practitioner will check the general state of health of the patient and prescribe for this, as well as suggesting effective treatment for the ulcer itself.

For general remarks on treatment, see under Boils and Abscesses and try one of the suggested remedies. None, however, could be superior to Comfrey, because of its astonishing ability to aid cell proliferation, and thus heal the extensive sloughing and tissue damage characteristic of ulcers.

So this should be your first choice from herbal remedies.

Make a strong tea and apply it as a compress: or apply oil of Comfrey; or soothe come Comfrey ointment over the area.

Calendula - garden Marigold - is another famous healer to think of: use compresses of lotion made from the tincture, bandaged into place and renewed two or three times daily.

For a real grandmother remedy - and a remarkably effective one too - take a Cabbage leaf, wash it thoroughly, and dip it into boiling water to soften it, cut out the thick central rib, then wrap it round the ulcer and bandage it into place. It will draw out the poison - and will need to be thrown away and replaced quite often at first.

Washes of hot Sage, Thyme or Rosemary tea - a teaspoon infused, covered, in a cupful of boiling water for 10 minutes - will also help to combat infection.

A wash of cool Chamomile tea - infuse a teaspoon of the dried flower heads in a cupful of boiling water, covered, for 10 minutes, then strain and cool- will help soothe inflammation and pain.

See also Boils and Abscesses.

Varicose Veins

Those unsightly blue knots and bulges in the leg veins are due to a bottle-neck of blood, following weakening or collapse of the valves in deep veins and arteries. (Piles are another form of the same problem.) .

Constipation, certain conditions of the bladder or gynaecological problems can all put pressure on the arteries involved, as does excess weight and pregnancy, so any treatment should begin with a thorough medical check-up. Overhaul your diet at the same time to make sure that it supplies plenty of fibre from vegetables, fruit, wholegrains; the fibre in some fruits will also supply bioflavonoids, which help strengthen the walls of arteries, veins and capillaries.

People often prefer to blame their varicose veins on heredity, but even if they're right, there's plenty you can do to make sure that an inherited tendency doesn't develop into a real problem. Even if some of your veins are already varicosed and the valves collapsed beyond repair, you can still do a lot to ginger up your circulation, strengthen the walls of veins, arteries and the tiniest capillaries, and stop the condition getting any worse. Surgical treatment of the problem is tempting if one or two veins are particularly unsightly, but if you have surgery you should realise that closing off one vein inevitably puts an extra workload on another, so redouble preventive care at the same time. Some of the commonest causes of varicose veins are:

Constipation - especially if it encourages you to spend hours on the loo straining, while deep in a book or the morning paper. If this is your problem, see under Constipation.

Smoking is a major factor, since it reduces the supply of oxygen to the blood. So is pregnancy.

Sitting a long time in a lovely hot bath. If this is a luxury you can't resist, at least do your legs the kindness of showering them with a jet of ice-cold water at the end, and rubbing them briskly with the roughest towel you have.

Standing about for hours on end - policemen and shop assistants are often victims. Sitting about all day is just as bad particularly if you sit slumped. The powerful muscles of the calf help pump blood up and down your legs, and a good brisk regular walk - at the very least - will help to keep them functioning efficiently.

Sitting with one leg crossed over the other constricts the circulation at knee-level. If you consciously make an effort to correct this deplorable habit, you'll have the pleasure of noticing that almost everyone else around you is still indulging in it.

The specific herbal remedy for varicose veins is a substance called Rutin, excellent for the strengthening of veins and capillaries. It's found in rose-hips, grapes, blackcurrants and citrus fruits, but by far the richest source is Buckwheat. You can buy Rutivite Tablets made from 100 per cent pure Buckwheat, compressed into tablet form. Dissolve three of them in a pint of boiling water and allow to stand for 10 minutes to make a pale yellowish-green tea, to be drunk three times a day, a cupful at a time; or you can add a tablet to your pot of tea. Either way the flavour is a little odd, but you will probably get used to it. Alternatively, you can swallow the tablets whole; take Rutivite 'E' in capsule form, with added

Vitamin E, or you can buy Rutin Tablets from many herbal suppliers. Rutin and Vitamin E, incidentally, will lessen your chances of suffering from high blood pressure, if you take them regularly.

To relieve the aching pain of varicose veins, compresses of Witch Hazel, or Tincture of Calendula, or a mixture- of the two, bandaged lightly round your legs and left on all night if possible, will help.

If you're varicose veins start getting worse, or give you a lot of pain, seek expert advice.

Warts & Verrucas

The cutting or burning out of warts and verrucas is getting less and less popular with doctors, since it doesn't seem to stop them recurring. They're caused by a virus, and appear to be associated with a temporary weakness of the body's immune system - which might perhaps explain' why psychological treatment or 'charming' them away often works wonders. So can simple herbal remedies - try one of these:

Paint them twice a day with strong vinegar in which the rinds of two Lemons have been macerated for eight days. Crush a clove of Garlic and apply it in a fresh poultice at night-time; protect the surrounding skin with sticking plaster. Repeat until the wart or verruca shows signs of disappearing. Rub the wart or verruca with a cut Onion, and leave the juice to dry on it. Paint with fresh Lemon juice, or soak the lint in the middle of a sticking plaster with Lemon juice and strap it on.

An old gipsy remedy is the milky juice squeezed from the stem of a Dandelion. Even in mid-city, there's usually a patch of waste land with the odd Dandelion growing on it somewhere. The milky juice will harden into a film – keep painting more on till the wart darkens and falls off.

Paint on Tincture of Thuja, from a homoeopathic chemist.

See also Bunions, Corns and Feet.

Children's Ailments

The usual range of children's ailments - fevers, colds, chills, cuts and. grazes,' sore throats, sleeping problems – can normally be dealt with from a very small range of gentle but effective herbs, of which Chamomile - for sleeplessness, upset tummies, nightmares - Lime Flowers, for restlessness, nausea - and Lemon Balm, for fevers, are the outstanding examples. The Spanish would add a fourth: Lemon Verbena, as mild as these and used by them as an all-purpose remedy for childish complaints. They call it *Hierba Luisa.* Lemon Balm and Lemon Verbena are easily grown in the garden, or in pots on your kitchen windowsill: keep teabags of Chamomile and Lime Flowers at hand. Normally healthy babies and children will respond to even small doses of these herbs, and the dose should be calculated according to age and size. If a grownup needs a cupful, a ten-year-old will need only a small glassful, a toddler a tablespoon or two, and a baby just a little to sip now and again from a bottle. (The exception is, of course, diarrhoea or fever, in both of which fluid intake should be as high as possible: so make a weaker infusion and give more).

Before tackling skin, digestive, nervous or respiratory problems, read the section on Allergies, and pause to consider the possibility. Thousands of children today are regularly dosed with antibiotics, sedatives', steroids or aspirin for conditions that would clear rapidly if suspect foods or chemicals were removed. Artificial food colourings have been implicated in hyperactivity in babies, as well as nervous or behavioural problems in older children, so you would be well advised to ban from your home foodstuffs contaminated with these needless chemicals - bottled fruit squashes, hundreds of tinned or processed foodstuffs, preserved meats, even syrups commonly given to babies. Check labels carefully. Fortunately, many supermarkets now do their best for mothers concerned about such additives: Safeway announced last year that they were removing all artificial food colouring from their entire range of own-label products.

Children eating a healthy diet and getting plenty of fresh air and exercise will seldom need more than the gentle herbal remedies suggested in this section, and as your own skill and expertise at coping with minor problems develops over the' years, you may well find that they never need to go to the doctor at all. But major illness can develop with frightening speed in small children, and I have indicated where appropriate the occasions when you should send for professional help without delay.

Acne

For general advice, see Acne. The time to nip this teenage agony in the bud is when the very first tiny pimples appear.

Cutting out sweets, chocolate, fried or rich foods, and eating lots of salads, all the brightly coloured vegetables - carrots, peppers, parsley, spinach, broccoli which are rich in betacarotene - may clear the condition without further treatment: explain to the sufferer that it's up to him or her to be sensible about their food for this reason. More stubborn cases can be helped by a professional herbal practitioner.

Asthma

See the sections on Asthma and Allergies generally. When young children are asthmatic, it's particularly important to track down the allergens which are causing this condition: with sound medical direction, and care on your part, they should grow out of it to enjoy a normal healthy childhood.

Allergies

Babies and growing children alike need all the excellent nutrients which are so abundantly supplied in whole wheat and dairy products such as milk, cheese and yogurt. If you or any member of the family discovers that they are allergic to either of these two basic food groups, it's important to get professional advice on how to make up the nutritional deficit.

This is particularly vital in the case of children: doctors today are seeing cases of actual malnutrition brought about by well-meaning parents attempting to sort out an allergic problem on their own.

See also Allergies

Bed Wetting

When a child old enough to know better - over four or five – is still wetting his bed at night, either he can't help it, in which case there may be a physical problem which your family doctor should investigate, or he's trying to tell you something, Either way, scolding won't help, and could turn a quite minor, if annoying, problem into a major psychological struggle, Try to make bedtime extra soothing and reassuring, with lots of hugs and cuddles, and if the bed is occasionally wet in the morning, don't make a fuss. Keep his diet plain and sensible, and see that he gets plenty of fresh air and exercise. The problem may be a deficiency of calcium and magnesium: milk and cheese are good sources of calcium, and nuts, fruit and vegetables of magnesium - especially dark green leafy vegetables like spinach. The wrong diet, high in refined foods and additives, can produce an irritable bladder, and bed wetting. The problem may also be one consequence of a food allergy: milk, eggs and citrus fruits are common culprits. If the condition is persistent, try removing these foods from the child's diet for four or five days, and see if matters improve.

See section on Allergies.

After checking his peace of mind - and his diet – try any of the following suggestions. Keep liquid intake low in the few hours before bedtime.

A small bedtime drink of hot milk sweetened with a teaspoon of honey, into which you stir a good pinch of Cinnamon.

Take equal parts of St John's Wort and Plantain Leaves. Infuse a teaspoonful in a cup of boiling water, sweeten with honey, and give it a little at a time throughout the day, with a last dose at bedtime. These healing herbs will soothe an irritated bladder. St John's Wort on its own is also effective.

It's one of the many useful herbs packaged in handy teabag form in the Greither's Floradix range.

Corn Silk - the tassels from ears of Sweet Corn - is also useful in easing inflammation or irritation of the urinary tract.

Make an infusion, sweeten with honey and give it as above.

See also Sleeplessness in Babies and Small Children.

Burns - *see page 44*

Colds and Coughs and Chestiness

For colds in babies or very small children, give infusions of the mildest herbs: Lemon Balm, Catnip, Chamomile. Give small drinks, keeping the child well covered up. Give lots of fruit juice, diluted with spring water, or plain spring water. A drop or two of the essential oil of Eucalyptus, put on their pillow or on a tissue tucked under their pillow, will often clear a cold overnight. For that nasty stuffy feeling, I used to give my children a 'sniffer' - a hanky with a few drops of Olba's Oil on it, to keep under their pillow and sniff at from time to time.

They loved, too, the fuss of a Mustard foot-bath, to be resorted to at the very first signs of chills or sniffs. Take a plastic bucket, put a couple of heaped spoonfuls of mustard powder in it - I add a tablespoon of ordinary washing soda too, since our London tap water is very hard - and then pour on enough hot water to come above the ankles, whisking briskly to mix it all. The child sits with his feet in this for about 10 minutes - top the water up from time to time to keep it nice and hot. Then-towel his feet dry, put on thick socks, and straight to bed. After this dose of a potent natural antibiotic, there will often be no trace of cold or cough the following morning.

'Elderflower Tea is particularly suitable for childish coughs and colds: put a teaspoonful of the dried flowers in a cup, fill it up with boiling water, cover and leave to infuse for twenty minutes. Sweeten with a little honey. If you have any Peppermint, add a couple of leaves, or half a teaspoon of the dried herb. Give this at bedtime, and cover the child up warmly.

Another excellent remedy for coughs is made by slicing three or four fine fat cloves of Garlic, and leaving them to 'marinate' for a few hours in half a cup of honey. Children will quite cheerfully swallow teaspoon-doses of the odd but quite pleasant runny liquid that results: give it every two to three hours. Very effective.

For the chesty coughs of children, Weleda' s Herb & Honey

Elixir is so delicious that they'll be eager to get to the next dose: not surprising, since it contains quantities of sugar and honey. It also contains glycerine, to help coat the throat with the Marshmallow, Icelandic Moss, White Horehound, Aniseed, Elder Flower and Thyme in it, which will help counter infection, inflammation and mild fever, as well as taking the edge off the cough with remarkable speed. A good soothing middle-of-the-night remedy. (But urge the child to brush teeth like mad the following morning ....) Potter's E.P.C. - fiery red stuff - combines Elderflowers and Peppermint with other herbs that give the circulation a healthy shot in the arm. For children from about five, give a teaspoon in a glass of warm water, preferably at bedtime. The mere sight of the bottle has been known to stop our children's colds in their tracks!

Colic in Babies

Colic in tiny babies usually indicates an allergic problem: often to the milk in-his formula, or the cereal, egg or other solid food in his diet. Even breastfed babies can react in this way to allergens of which their mother's milk still contains traces.

Treat by removing the suspect foods from his diet for a few days to see if the condition clears, then let a long time go by before you try the same food on him again - when he may have no reaction at all.

Meanwhile, to ease the pain and discomfort, give teaspoon doses of a tea made from Fennel Seeds or Caraway Seeds from time to time. Dill seeds are another well known remedy for baby colic. They're used in the Gripe Water which some mothers find as delicious as it's effective.

Crush a teaspoon of the Dill, Fennel or Caraway seeds and steep them in a cupful of boiling water, covered, for twenty minutes, then strain off Catmint or Chamomile tea, infused covered, are both mild and effective remedies for a baby's digestive discomfort.

Constipation

Constipation in children should be corrected first and foremost by seeing that their diet supplies plenty of the natural fibre in fruit, vegetables and whole grains, that they get enough exercise, and that they go to the lavatory as soon as they feel the urge. Apples are particularly useful for clearing up constipation. If the condition persists, consult a herbal practitioner. It is not advisable to start children on the laxative habit.

Convalescence

Like grownups, children need time for their bodies to get over the stress of illness. There's no need to cosset them too much, but by the same token don't rush them back to school or busy everyday life, if they're still looking pale and peaky. Keep their diet simple, with plenty of fruit and raw vegetables, or nourishing soups: give them bottled spring water or fruit juices to drink. See that they get lots of sleep, with a bedtime drink of Chamomile tea to make it deep and refreshing.

Two excellent herbal tonics are, first, Bio-Strath Elixir: see Convalescence and Kindervital by Floradix, a popular German product. Both are packed with herbal goodness to stimulate jaded appetites, promote growth, soothe the nervous system and supply needed nutrients. Since Kindervital contains Vitamin D derived from yeast, it should not be taken at the same time as extra Vitamin D prescribed by the doctor.

Among the herbs it contains are spices like Coriander and Aniseed, soothing Liquorice Root, Fennel to help clear mucus and calcium and Vitamin D to help build healthy bones.

Cuts, Grazes, and Scratches

When there are small children around the house, first aid for badly grazed knees, cuts, and scratches will always be in demand, and the four remedies I would never be without are Weleda's Tincture of Calendula - soothing, healing and antiseptic;

Nelson's Tincture of Hypercal, for really severe cases – it combines Calendula with the marvellous painkilling and healing properties of Hypericum - St John's Wort; a soft Comfrey Ointment, and Calendula Ointment.

Very bad grazes, with dirt or gravel imbedded in them, should be swabbed gently with pieces of cotton wool soaked in plenty of hand-hot (boiled) water to which you have added half a teaspoonful of Tincture of Calendula. Throwaway each piece of cotton wool after using it once. If possible soak the grazed part till the dirt seems to have come out. Then dress it with a piece of gauze wrung out in more warm water with a few drops of added Calendula, put clean lint on top, and bandage into place. After a day or two you can take off the dressing and let it heal swiftly on its own. If it does not heal quickly, and pus comes out, soak off the first dressing with more warm water and Calendula, and re-dress.

Cuts and scratches can be dealt with in the same way. For smaller ones, put a little Calendula Ointment onto the gauze in a sticking plaster, or wash them with Calendula lotion and leave to heal on their own, unless they're likely to get dirt in them during an afternoon in the garden or playground.

When the graze is particularly painful, Comfrey Ointment is soothing. When children are reluctant to let you touch a sore spot, as they often are, they're quite happy to spread a timid fingerful of this on the hurt themselves. Garlic Ointment: another fine antiseptic. (They used Garlic dressings at the Front during World War I, to prevent bad wounds becoming gangrenous.)

Any of these treatments will guarantee fast natural healing with a minimum of scarring.

If you don't have any of these remedies, honey is an excellent cooling and antiseptic treatment.

Diarrhoea in Children and Babies

In babies and small children, acute diarrhoea is always a case for a doctor - dehydration and collapse can happen with frightening speed. Keep the child warm meanwhile, and give it a sip of weak Chamomile tea, or warm water with a little honey added. A hand-hot compress of Chamomile tea on the baby's stomach will help relieve the pain. Other remedies for mild cases:

Meadowsweet tea: made by pouring a cupful of almost boiling water' over a teaspoonful of the herb, then steeping, covered, for ten minutes. Add a little honey. It should be drunk as warm as possible.

Chamomile tea: A teaspoonful of the flower heads steeped for ten minutes in a cupful of hot water. It should be drunk warm.

Catnip tea: A teaspoonful in a cupful of boiling water. Steep, covered, for twenty minutes. If you have none of these herbs, chop up one big Onion and infuse it, covered, in a litre (1 ½ pint) of boiling water for two hours. Sweeten with a little honey. Give a spoonful from time to time.

Honey, be recommended for infantile diarrhoea since it contains small amount of vital mineral salts - particularly potassium – which need to be replaced fast in this condition.

Grated raw apple: The pectin content helps it to absorb the contents of the bowel and ease their passage.

Weleda's Melissa Compound. Five to ten drops in water every four hours will also help. It contains soothing Lemon Balm, Angelica to warm and relax the stomach, and Clove, Nutmeg, Coriander, Cinnamon and Lemon. Virtually tasteless, it's a particularly easy remedy to give children.

Slippery Elm Root is comforting and nourishing. Mix a teaspoonful of the powder to a paste with a little cold water, and then pour boiling water on, stirring hard. Add Cinnamon and a little honey.

When the child is over the worst, keep the diet specially simple and plain for the next two or three days, and if they don't feel hungry, a day or two without food other than Slippery Elm will do them no harm at all. When they feel hungry again, plain boiled whole rice, purees of lightly cooked vegetables - particularly carrots - and mashed ripe bananas with a little yogurt are all excellent. Bottled spring water should replace fruit juice and fizzy drinks, and sweets, chocolate, sugar and fruit other than bananas should be avoided.

Digestive Upsets
Excitement, apprehension, too many sweets or rich party food, all can play havoc with a child's digestion. Sipping warm water

often helps all by itself: for bad cases, add peace and calm and bed. Chamomile or Peppermint Tea is calming and soothing. To allay pain, Slippery Elm is very effective. If they feel sick, encourage them to vomit, if possible. A pinch of dried ginger added to Chamomile or Peppermint tea will counter nausea.

See also Digestive Problems, and read the section on Allergies. If digestive upsets are recurrent, seek professional help.

Earache

It's particularly important to get professional help fast for earache in children, since untreated it can develop very quickly into a serious problem, causing intense pain. Meanwhile, use the emergency measures suggested in the adult section on Earache. If, however, your child has a perforated ear drum, no drops should be put into the ear: instead, simply put the Garlic oil, Mullein oil or Lemon juice on a piece of sterilised and warmed cotton wool, tuck it just inside the ear, and wrap a scarf around the head to keep it in place.

Eczema

Often dismissed by doctors as one of those passing childhood problems, to be treated - if at all- with steroid creams, eczema almost invariably signals a food allergy, with milk as usual the prime suspect. Try taking milk out of the diet for four or five days: you can substitute one of the unsweetened soybean milks from a health food store meanwhile. If the eczema clears, you'll know you're on the right track: then you need professional help planning a healthy milk-free diet for your child. If it doesn't clear, check the diet for other possible allergens. Vitamin B deficiencies can also cause eczema: so try adding a little wheat germ to cereals. See also Eczema in the adult section.

A deficiency in essential fatty acids is another possible cause: many cases of infantile eczema clear up rapidly if the child is given half to two teaspoons of pure Sunflower or

Safflower oil a day. If the deficiency is not corrected by pure vegetable oils, try Oil of Evening Primrose (see adult section).

For babies it may be enough simply to smooth the oil into the affected parts, or rub it into the soft crook of the elbow.

The child still has eczema? Seek expert advice. Your family doctor will probably prescribe corticosteroid creams. These will certainly clear the eczema with gratifying speed, but they may not resolve the underlying problem, and they can do long-term damage to your child's developing immune system, so be cautious about using them.

The dry scaling skin of infantile eczema usually worries parents much more than it bothers the actual sufferer. But if it's itchy and sore, bathe the affected parts in a lotion made by adding half a teaspoon of Tincture of Calendula to a cupful of boiled, distilled or bottled spring water.

Or make a strong infusion of Chamomile from a handful of the dried flower heads steeped for twenty minutes in a pint of boiling water, covered; add it to the baby's bedtime bath.

Or make up some of Weleda's Eczema Tea, and add it to the bath.

Fevers and Infectious Diseases
The fevers of childhood ailments can be alarming to an inexperienced mother, particularly as a child's temperature can climb with frightening speed. In such cases, it's better to err on the side of caution: call the doctor without delay.

Meanwhile, put the patient to bed in a well-ventilated room, in clean pyjamas or nightie, and give any of the following mild herbal infusions, which will relax and calm while gently assisting the beneficial action of the fever. Lime Flower, Catmint, Elder Flower or Lemon Balm - whichever you have to hand - can all be made up into a hot infusion: use a heaped teaspoon of the fresh herb, or rather less of the dried, to a cupful of boiling water, and infuse for ten minutes. Any of these will be particularly useful at the start of a fever, and you can give one of them to your child while you wait for the doctor. For children under two, a small medicine glassful will be enough: for children up to ten, half a wineglassful. These teas should be given three times a day. In between, give plenty of spring water or diluted fruit drinks. Don't urge food on children in the early stages of fevers or infectious diseases: they're unlikely to be hungry in any case. When they are hungry again, keep food light and simple: chicken soup, finger salads, plenty of fresh fruit.

Most of the childhood infectious diseases - mumps, chicken pox, German measles and so on - run their course with very little trouble for anyone beyond a mild fever and a rash. But Measles needs particularly good nursing care from you, because it can be a dangerous illness with unpleasant complications: it seems to make its victims extraordinarily vulnerable to other infections - pneumonia and eye infections among them. Diet should be kept light, with plenty of fruit juice and any of the following herbs, infused and drunk hot:

Elder Flowers, Yarrow, Peppermint, sweetened if liked with a little honey; infuse a teaspoonful in a cup of boiling water, and give half a cupful three times a day. Don't flood the sickroom with light in the case of measles, as the eyes seem to be particularly susceptible to infection. If they become sore, see under Conjunctivitis for treatment, remembering how important scrupulous cleanliness is. Call the doctor again at the first sign of any serious complications.

Many children sail through Chickenpox, with hardly a single pustule to prove they've got it, but others are driven nearly mad with irritation by their little itchy blisters. Give them calming Lime Flower tea - use the teabags which even supermarkets and delicatessens sell these days, and treat the blisters with any of the remedies suggested in the section on Shingles, which is caused by the same virus.

For Whooping Cough seek expert advice immediately.

Always a disagreeable illness in children, whooping cough can threaten the lives of small babies, since it can lead to pneumonia, while the massive inflammation of the lungs can produce lasting scarring, leaving them impaired in function, and the child permanently vulnerable to bronchial infection.

Like Measles, too, whooping cough leaves its victims especially susceptible to other infections. Careful nursing is needed as much during convalescence as in the acute stage of the illness.

Even if your family doctor prescribes a course of powerful modern antibiotics, you can safely administer any of the following aromatic plants as well. Used in ways that allow their healing and antiseptic volatile oils to penetrate deep into the lungs, they can certainly help your child throw off whooping cough and make a steady recovery.

A hot infusion of common-or-garden Thyme. Steep a small teaspoonful or a small sprig, covered, in boiling water for 10 minutes. Sweeten it with plenty of honey, and give the child a tablespoonful three times a day - or for a baby, a little in a bottle.

Garlic is powerfully bactericidal, as dozens of folk remedies for respiratory disease all around the world testify. An easy way to administer it to a child is to slice up several cloves of Garlic, put them in a small jar, cover them with two or three tablespoons of honey, and let them stand for three to four hours. At the end of this time, the honey will have turned into a thin runny liquid which doesn't taste nearly as strong as you might expect. Give the child a teaspoonful every four hours or so. Garlic Ointment or Garlic Oil squeezed out of a capsule can be rubbed into the chest and back or the soles of the feet, for babies. Like all aromatic plants, the volatile oil of Garlic is highly diffusible, and after rapid absorption through the skin, it circulates through the bloodstream to be eliminated via the lungs.

In French aromatherapy, the essential oil of Cypress is considered a specific for the treatment of whooping cough.

You can buy the Essential Oil of Cypress from Neal's Yard Apothecary. Put a few drops on the patient's pillow from time to time.

For drinks, give Chamomile tea, sweetened with honey. It calms the spasms of whooping cough, is mildly sedative and very soothing.

Lemon Balm or Catnip tea, both made with a teaspoon of the fresh or dried leaves in a cupful of boiling water, infused, tightly covered, for ten minutes, then strained and sweetened with honey, are also good for calming and soothing a restless, feverish child. For small babies, give a teaspoonful at a time, making sure that it's not too hot, or put it in a bottle. Children can be given a small cupful to sip three times a day.

After the worst of the .illness is over, patients need a good tonic to help restore their strength and vitality: see under Convalescence. Particularly suitable for small children: Slippery Elm, Bio-Strath Elixir and Royal Jelly are all good strengthening tonics for a child recovering from whooping cough.

After any of these infectious illnesses, or a fever accompanied by one of those inexplicable rashes which seem to be becoming more common, children need time to recover and build up their strength again. See Convalescence.

Headaches

If these are severe or persistent, you need professional advice. They can also be due to a food Allergy - milk, eggs, chocolate and wheat are common offenders - in which case a little detective work On your part may identify it, and help you clear up a tendency to fatigue and irritability at the same time: these are both common allergic symptoms in children. But children's headaches - particularly the kind that come on suddenly – are often due to a digestive upset, caused by too much rich food, or even chemical additives. If this is the case, there is usually a degree of nausea, often relieved by vomiting. A drink of warm water may bring this on, after which the child will feel much better. Put the sufferer to bed in a darkened room (remove books and comics to forestall temptation!) arid give them a cup of Lime Flower or Chamomile tea. Cold compresses of Witch Hazel on their forehead are very comforting. Sleep is often the most effective cure.

Head lice

Help for the ubiquitous head lice, to epidemics of which not even the snobbiest little private schools or playgroups seem immune, and which are often attracted to the cleanest, shiniest long hair in the school. The treatment smells a lot nicer than the vile proprietary preparation usually recommended by schools, and at the end of the treatment, she reports, 'not only were my children completely lice-free but they were the owners of lustrous, shining healthy hair'. To make up the treatment, you need four Essential Oils: 25 drops of Rosemary, 12 drops Eucalyptus, 13 drops Geranium, and 25 drops Lavender, in 3fl oz's of vegetable oil. Section the hair from the forehead to the neck and saturate it with the oil right down to the roots, section by section. If the child has long hair, pile it on top of the head, and make sure every bit is oiled. Then wrap cling-film right round the head, behind the ears and covering all the hair (but do be careful not to let it anywhere near nose and mouth, for obvious reasons). Leave on for a couple 'of hours, then take off over the bath. Add shampoo and rub it well in, then rinse thoroughly, and comb through with a fine nit-comb. Repeat three days later.

Hyperactivity, irritability and nervous problems

Hyperactivity in babies is fast becoming a modern epidemic, which few doctors are experienced in coping with. In the' full blown form of this distressing problem, babies are perpetually irritable, cry for hours on end, often sleep only an hour or two at a time, and generally destroy all peace of mind, calm and relaxation for the luckless families into which they are born. This degree ~ hyperactivity can have multiple causes - from heavy metal/ intoxication to food or chemical sensitivities - see Allergies - but the colouring in processed foods is a common culprit (used in plenty of fruit drinks for babies and small children, and in the very medicine doctors most frequently recommend for the condition). So as a first step, eliminate all trace of colouring matter from the diet, which should be as simple, healthy and .nutritious as possible.

Improvement in the diet, together with regular brisk exercise and plenty of fresh air, will often clear the condition and strengthen the nervous system by itself. Eliminate tea, coffee, cocoa and chocolate as well as cola drinks, too, since these all contain caffeine which children are much better off without.

Some children are more temperamental and highly strung than others by nature, but tension, acute irritability, jumpiness, weepiness, regular inability to sleep, are all indications of a real problem, and a professional herbalist can prescribe herbs that will strengthen the whole nervous system, iron out tensions and calm frazzled nerves.

Mild remedies which will certainly help children with this kind of problem include Lime Flower or Vervain or Chamomile tea, all available in teabag form. Give them muesli for breakfast, soaked in water overnight, since Oats are wonderfully tonic to the nerves. Weleda's Avena Sativa is excellent for children as well as grownups: it contains Oats, plus calming sedative Hops, Passionflower and Valerian. For a calming bedtime bath, make a double-strength infusion of Lime Flowers, and slip it into the bath.

But no child, however temperamental or highly strung by nature, should need treatment of this kind more than once in a while, so if these simple measures fail to clear it, consult a herbal practitioner who will get to the root of the problem.

Nappy Rash

Use a soothing and healing ointment- Comfrey, Calendula or Marshmallow.

If the baby's bottom is very red and sore, make up a pint of an infusion of Chamomile Flowers or Elder Flowers, allow it to cool, and apply a gauze pad wrung out in it to the most painful parts.

A teaspoonful of Tincture of Calendula or Tincture of Hypericum added to a glassful of cold boiled water can be used in the same way, between changes of nappy. Exposure to fresh air is usually the best cure - though not always practicable.

See also Eczema, Sleeplessness in Babies, Skin Problems

Sleeplessness

Sleeplessness in babies and small children may be due simply to the need for hugs and reassurance, for which no herbal remedy can possibly be a substitute. But to soothe that restless fractious crying, to calm mild digestive upsets, or to help at

Teething times, here are some safe and simple remedies.

The best of them all, which can safely be given even to small babies - as indeed can any of these - is Chamomile tea.

Alternatively, try Catnip tea. For both these remedies see Diarrhoea in Children and Babies.

Lemon Balm or Lemon Verbena, infused for ten minutes in a cupful of boiling water, are also safe and soothing.

For small babies, let the liquid cool a little and put a dessertspoonful in a feeding bottle. For older babies and small children, increase the dose up to half a cupful. All these teas can be sweetened with a little honey.

Weleda's Avena Sativa Compound is perfectly safe even for babies. Mix two to three drops in a little water.

If sleeplessness becomes chronic, night after night, there may be a real problem (see Hyperactivity) - or else the child has realised it's a super excuse for not getting off to bed quietly, and for an unfair share of grown-up attention.

See also Insomnia, Colic

Shock

Nasty tumbles, a visit to the dentist, scalds etc. can all produce quite serious states of shock in children. The best remedy I know is Dr Bach's Rescue Remedy (see Shock in adult section) together with plenty of hugs and reassurance.

Sore Throat

A remedy that will particularly appeal to children is Blackcurrant tea, made from a good jelly with no additives in it other than sugar and pectin, Put a heaped dessertspoonful in a cup, pour boiling water over it, add the juice of half a lemon, and a spot of honey if needed. When it has cooled a little, get the child to gargle with a little of it - holding it in their throat for as long as possible - and then drink the rest. Repeat three times a day.

Hot Sage or Thyme tea, made by infusing a teaspoon of the dried herb or more of the fresh in a cupful of boiling water, covered, for ten minutes, can also be used as a compress: dip a clean cotton scarf in the hot tea, wring it out, and wrap it round the throat; cover it with another scarf to keep it in place. See also adult section under Sore Throat.

Teething

Make up Calendula lotion by adding 5 drops of Tincture of Calendula to half a glass of boiled water: rub the gums gently with this. If the baby is fractious and can't sleep, soothing Chamomile or Lemon Balm tea will help. See under Sleeplessness.

Worms

The most common parasite found in human beings is the tiny threadworm, which settles into the intestines, and multiplies by crawling out to lay its eggs around the anus - usually at bedtime - which process· sets up a characteristic itching around the anus. Once thought to be a disease of the slums, worms are now rampant throughout the civilised world, and epidemics rage through every school from time to time, easily spread by unscrubbed fingernails that have scratched an itching bottom. In an attempt to contain the epidemic, most schools understandably insist that known cases be dealt with by a reliable drug: the standard one is Pripsen, bought in two dose sachets to be taken a fortnight apart - the length of the worm breeding cycle.

However, worms will only flourish in the right environment, which for them is an acid one, so if you drastically reduce sugar in the child's diet, and replace it by plenty of fruit, vegetables and whole grain cereals, you will discourage future infestations - not to mention improving your child's health.

Worms themselves have well known aversions to certain foods - particularly Garlic and Onions, raw Carrots, Pumpkin seeds. Plenty of these should be eaten, and to deliver them on target, first thing in the morning. Pumpkin seeds can be ground in a coffee grinder, and added to breakfast muesli.

Garlic or Onion infusions, to be drunk first thing in the morning: grate a small Onion, or slice3or4 cloves of Garlic into a mug, pour a cupful of boiling water over them, cover, and leave to steep overnight.

A famous peasant cure for worms is to stick a clove of Garlic up the anus every night for a fortnight. Much .less uncomfortable, and just as effective: a thin smear of Garlic Ointment around the anus, every night for a fortnight.

See also Sprains and Fractures, Tonsillitis, Toothache, Warts and Verrucas.